NUTRITION IN THE WOMB

NUTRITION IN THE WOMB

*How better nutrition during development
will prevent heart disease, diabetes and stroke*

The Developmental Origins of Health and Disease (DOHAD):
a call for action by

DAVID BARKER MD

Cover and text design: Anita Jones, Another Jones Graphics
Cover illustrations: Fred Harwin, Fred Harwin Studios

Barker, D. J. P. (David James Purslove)
        Nutrition in the womb : how better nutrition during
    development will prevent heart disease, diabetes and
    stroke : The developmental origins of health and disease
    (DOHAD): a call for action / by David
    Barker. -- 1st ed.
        p. cm.
        LCCN 2008904567
        ISBN-13: 978-09816449-0-5
        ISBN-10: 09816449-0-2

        1. Pregnancy--Nutritional aspects. 2. Mothers--
    Nutrition. 3. Nutritionally induced diseases.
    I. Title.

    RG559.B375 2008   618.2'42
                                 QBI08-600157

Printed in the USA

A portion of the proceeds from the sale of this book shall go to the Barker Foundation, a non-profit organization established in Oregon to improve nutrition in the womb.

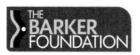

www.TheBarkerFoundation.org

CONTENTS

1   Heart Attack   1

2   Heart Attacks Begin in the Womb   11

3   Low Birthweight Increases the Risk
of Heart Disease   17

4   The Malnourished Baby   23

5   Why the Malnourished Baby has a
Less Healthy Life   39

6   Mothers' Diets   53

7   Mothers' Bodies   79

8   Infants Who Fail to Thrive   97

9   Children Who Grow Differently   119

10   Adults Who Had Low Birthweight   141

11   Pathways to Health at all Ages   157

FOREWORD

ONE OF THE most famous quotes in American history is that "All men are created equal." It is the basis of democracy in the U.S. and has helped to shape the country. Ironically, not all babies are created equal. A baby's chance of surviving and living a healthy life is influenced significantly by the mother's nutrition.

We have known for a long time that the nutrition of the mother can have a profound effect on the fetus and newborn. Early work of Agnes Higgins showed that providing food supplements to pregnant women improved diet quality and birth outcomes. The 1969 White House Conference on Food, Nutrition and Health observed that "food supplementation of high risk pregnant women and their infants was warranted." This recommendation paved the way for the creation of the Special Supplemental Food Program for Women, Infants and Children (WIC). Evaluations from the WIC Program document the positive impact of nutritious food supplements in decreasing low birth weight. Studies from around the world (Narangwal, Tamil Nadu, the Gambia) have observed similar positive effects of food supplements for high risk pregnant women.

However, we now know even more. Dr. David Barker's ground breaking research has irrevocably influenced the way in which the medical and nutrition community now views optimal development. In this book *Nutrition in the Womb* the author elucidates the complex linkages between a woman's nutrition prior to and during pregnancy and the health of her child for decades to come. Children born small have a significantly higher risk of developing chronic diseases in mid-life. If we are to reverse the burgeoning rates of obesity, diabetes, and heart diseases new paradigms for nutrition programs and policies must be employed. The nutrition architecture needs to emphasize prevention and invest in females before they become pregnant. Regrettably, rarely have the classic nutrition programs been able to reach girls prior to pregnancy. This book tells us how to be more effective. *Nutrition in the Womb* takes the reader beyond discovery.

In a clear, concise format, the book summarizes the large volume of research defining the links between early nutrition and the risk of later chronic disease. More importantly, this book answers the question, "So What?" *Nutrition in the Womb* is a must read book for anyone interested in promoting health and wellness. Investing in the nutrition of our children now is imperative for promoting healthy lives for generations to come.

Eileen Kennedy, D.Sc.
Dean, Friedman School of Nutrition Science and Policy
Tufts University
March, 2008

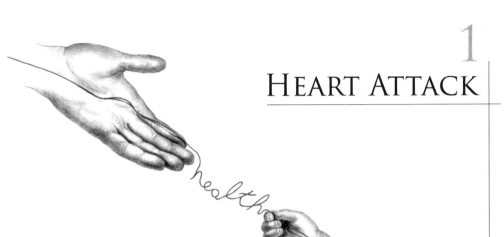

HEART ATTACK

WE ARE WITNESSES TO A DISASTER. Coronary heart disease was almost unknown a hundred years ago. Now it is the most common cause of death in the world. There is a rising epidemic of diabetes, which causes heart disease. Soon 250 million people will have diabetes. Patients are told that they are sick because of the way they live. When they reply that they live like others, who are healthy, they are told their genes are at fault. When they ask which genes, no-one knows. When they ask how genes could cause an epidemic, there is no reply. Motor cars break down for two reasons. Either they are driven on rough roads, or they are badly put together. If they are well made they can be driven on any road. The body is no different. Chronic disease can be prevented by improving the growth and development of babies. This book presents the evidence.

> *Chronic disease can be prevented by improving the growth and development of babies.*

HEART ATTACK

For several months he had felt short of breath and had had tightness in his chest. He passed these off as the result of lack of exercise and indigestion. He was an unusually energetic man, who maintained a demanding seven day a week schedule, an exercise enthusiast, a man with proven ability to withstand prolonged and exceptional stress. Regular six monthly medical check-ups over many years had revealed nothing untoward except slightly raised blood pressure and cholesterol. On the day he walked into the emergency room in a New York hospital he felt well. His visit to hospital was merely a precaution. He was shocked when x-rays showed that ninety percent of the arteries supplying blood to the muscles of his heart were blocked. So too were his family when they were told he needed immediate surgery. He was in danger and could suffer a major heart attack at any time.

At a press conference his wife said "my husband's optimism and faith will carry him through the difficult weeks and months ahead, of that we have no doubt." His daughter stood silently by. Over the next week he received 45,000 letters. A typical one read, "You are surrounded by cherished friends and a nation that adores you and prays for your full and complete recovery."

During surgery they stopped his heart. The surgeons removed the extensive blockages. Newspapers and magazines described every detail of the operation and every stage of his recovery. "So why," they asked, "did our former president come so close to death?"; for the patient was Bill Clinton.

The press, advised by medical experts across the country, blamed his bad diet for the blockages in his arteries. They wrote about his life-long liking for fatty foods. "All those saturated fats and that cholesterol from burgers and tacos and barbecued ribs went not just to Clinton's waist but into his blood as well. And those fats built up into fatty deposits known as plaques that slowly but surely massed within the walls of his arteries" wrote Time magazine.

It is fashionable to attribute coronary heart disease to the food people eat. But evidence to support this is seriously lacking. If there was solid evidence that the tens of thousands of Americans who die each year of heart disease are the victims of junk food; if it was junk food that almost killed the President; then surely these foods should be withdrawn. If pizza is that lethal someone should mention it to the Italians. When a mayonnaise was recently found to contain bacteria which killed five people the product was immediately taken off the shelves.

> *It is fashionable to attribute coronary heart disease to the food people eat. But evidence to support this is seriously lacking.*

The ever-changing advice given to the public about which foods are good and which are bad reveals a lack of secure scientific knowledge. Milk is bad for you: milk is good for you. Beef will kill you: beef makes you strong. Do not eat eggs: eat eggs. How many eggs? One a week; no two; no three. To put the blame for heart disease on the junk food people eat is not wholly wrong, and everyone who promotes good health advocates a good diet. But as an explanation for the most common cause of death in the world it is seriously incomplete. To begin with it does not take into account what each of us knows from our own observations. Many people who live on hamburgers and fries do not get heart disease. Nor does it explain why the disease increases rapidly in countries as they westernise. And nor does it explain why, within a country, there is more of the disease in one place than in another.

> *The ever-changing advice given to the public about which foods are good and which are bad reveals a lack of secure scientific knowledge.*

The former President needed his operation because the walls of the arteries supplying blood to the muscle of his heart had become hardened, and the channels within them narrowed by deposits of fat. Hardening of the arteries is part of the history of mankind. It was found in the arteries of Egyptian mummies and in the arteries of a man buried in the ice 5000 years ago. Until 100 years ago,

Something more than hardening of the arteries must be happening. Something related to westernisation and fatty deposits in arteries. Something catastrophic.

however, heart attacks were uncommon. They appeared in western countries and increased so rapidly that within fifty years they had become the most common cause of death. Today there are similar rising epidemics in the third world, in India, China and South America. 6 million people now die from heart disease each year. Something more than hardening of the arteries must be happening. Something related to westernisation and fatty deposits in arteries. Something catastrophic.

Fat, Fiber, Salt, Sugar, Meat: Which to Blame?

Fifty years ago, Ancel Keys, a nutritionist at the University of Minnesota, became aware that heart disease was common among business executives and other prosperous men. He could not understand why any disease would be common among well-nourished people. To investigate this he embarked on the now famous Seven Countries Study, in which he related the frequency of death from heart disease in each of seven countries to the diets of middle-aged men and women who lived there. He found that while death rates in the US were lower than those in Finland, they were twice as high as those in Italy, a finding that first popularized the Mediterranean diet as being healthy. But in the small island of Crete, to the south of Greece, death from coronary heart disease scarcely ever occurred. The rate in the US was an astonishing forty times higher.

The best-known finding in Keys' survey was that heart disease was more common in countries where people had higher levels of cholesterol in their blood. This link between raised cholesterol and heart disease has been confirmed many times since then, and drugs which lower cholesterol have been shown to reduce the risk of the disease. Because cholesterol is contained in fatty foods, Keys concluded that people who ate more fat were more at risk of heart disease. This has never been proved. Neither has it been possible to implicate any other single kind of food or nutrient.

Surprisingly there is no precise scientific definition of the word 'fat'. It is generally applied to foods that are obviously fatty in nature, greasy in texture and do not mix with water. Around the world foods that contain fat, such as meat and butter, tend to be lacking in the diets of poorer people, as they are expensive. As countries become wealthier more fat is consumed. Fats eaten in food are broken down by the body and used to manufacture essential substances, including cholesterol. Much of the cholesterol in the blood is manufactured by the body rather than eaten in food. Cholesterol is an important part of the walls or 'membranes' that form the barrier between one cell and another. For reasons that are not understood cholesterol is extremely important for animal cells, but plants do not use it. The cholesterol in our diet therefore comes almost entirely from animal foods.

Ancel Keys discovery of the link between the amount of cholesterol in the blood and the risk of heart disease seemed to be a major breakthrough that would allow us to control the epidemic. Since animal fats are the dietary source of the cholesterol in the blood, the argument ran, the disease would dwindle if we ate less fat. This has not been proved despite a massive investment of research resources. A direct link between how much fat a person eats and his or her risk of heart disease has proved impossible to establish. Doctors treating patients have become increasingly frustrated by the poor results of altering peoples' diets in an attempt to reduce the cholesterol levels in their blood, and hence reduce their risk of a heart attack.

A direct link between how much fat a person eats and his or her risk of heart disease has proved impossible to establish.

Nevertheless, and not unreasonably, public health programs were launched in the US to reduce consumption of animal fat. Older people rightly enquired why in their youth they had been advised to drink more milk to make them into healthier children, and now in middle life they were being instructed to drink less to prevent heart disease. Everywhere dairy industries were thrown into turmoil. Critics mocked "should every cow carry a government health warning?" The necessary scientific proof was lacking.

Then along came dietary fiber, borne on the wings of an old idea. In 1920, Rendle Short, a surgeon at the University of Bristol, England, published a paper. He was a devout man who wrote detailed accounts of the natural world as an act of thanks to the God who created them. Each year he chose a topic for his close inspection. One year he chose appendicitis, a disease that had previously been rare but was rising steeply to become one of the most common surgical emergencies in the western world. It killed young people; and it killed the children of the rich more often than it killed the children of the poor.

In his essay Rendle Short concluded that the epidemic of appendicitis had arisen as a result of "the relatively less quantity of cellulose (roughage) eaten on account of the wider use of imported foods". By eating less of the fiber in vegetables and coarse bread, people had slowed the passage of food through their bowels, which led to infections such as appendicitis. His essay led to an editorial in the Lancet, and to the marketing of a new breakfast cereal, All-Bran. The idea that acute appendicitis is caused by lack of fiber has failed to withstand the test of time. In the 1970s, however, lack of dietary fiber was reborn as an explanation for a whole group of diseases, including heart disease and diabetes. The makers of breakfast cereals popularized this idea. It too failed to withstand scientific scrutiny, but the idea lives on, and from it come huge profits.

People with hypertension (high blood pressure) are at risk of heart disease and may benefit from eating less salt. If the body retains too much salt, blood pressure rises. In the short term this happens because the fluid in the blood increases to dilute the salt. In the longer term, salt makes the walls of the arteries contract so that the arteries become narrowed. Do the people in the western world eat too much salt? Though a study of salt intake and blood pressure in 52 populations around the world gave only limited support to this, soon in restaurants and diners the salt pot was replaced by individual packs to prevent too much being added to food. Since most of the salt in our diets comes with the food we eat, especially processed foods, this was merely a symbolic gesture.

Finally, in the search for what could have triggered the heart disease epidemic attention turned to changes in consumption of particular foods. Was it the increasing availability of sugar in the US? Was it a fall in fish consumption? Was it the rising meat consumption of Americans, who now eat, on average, 72 grams of animal protein a day compared with a figure of around 10 grams in African countries? But nothing added up.

...in the search for what could have triggered the heart disease epidemic attention turned to changes in consumption of particular foods. But nothing added up.

As time passed, and heart disease continued to rise, the search for the culprit moved away from diet. Windscreen stickers proclaiming "butter kills" were no longer to be seen. The dairy industry was reprieved. Egg consumption rose. Another culprit had come into view. Smoking. In 1980 the link between smoking and heart disease was unclear. The link with lung cancer was clear, though the statement "smoking causes lung cancer" is only a partial truth. The full statement is "smoking causes lung cancer, in some smokers, and we do not know why some people are vulnerable while others are protected". As antismoking campaigns changed smoking habits, the people who continued to smoke were different to those who gave up. They differed in their diets, and in other aspects of their lifestyles. Smokers got more heart disease but how much of this was due to the smoke? It is not a question that requires an answer since there is wide agreement that smoking damages health and should be strongly discouraged. Exaggerated claims for the numbers of people whose heart disease was caused by cigarettes has diverted attention from key biological issues; and we still do not know what causes the most common fatal disease in the world.

...we still do not know what causes the most common fatal disease in the world.

The evidence that the lifestyles of men and women determine their risk of heart disease is not consistent. The disease is common among the vegetarian, non-smoking women of South India, and uncommon among the meat-eating, smoking men of southern France. For a non-smoking American man with a healthy diet and lifestyle, low blood pressure and low cholesterol, the most likely cause of death is still heart disease. Changes in people's lifestyles as adults do not explain the rising epidemics of coronary heart disease that are now occurring in the Third World.

The disease is common among the vegetarian non-smoking women of South India, and uncommon among the meat-eating, smoking men of southern France.

There have been trials in which thousands of people in the US improved their diets and lifestyles, for many months. The benefits have been disappointingly small, with only 8% fewer heart attacks at best. This and other disappointing results led the British Heart Foundation to conclude that, "We shall probably never have proof that a particular lifestyle factor or item of diet is important and those who demand proof before any action is taken are condemning us to wait forever." This is sensible. If there is a possibility that by changing peoples' lifestyles their chance of a heart attack can be reduced, or their slow descent into a life of heart failure, inability to walk, terrifying breathless nights, swollen ulcerated legs, can be arrested, who will not recommend it? Doctors are familiar with the need to advise patients in circumstances where there is only limited knowledge; and it is not the purpose of this book to undermine current advice about good lifestyles.

Unfortunately, however, the view that heart disease is simply the result of bad lifestyles has led people to conclude that a heart attack is the patient's fault. "If anyone had had bad habits", Time magazine wrote scathingly, "it was Bill Clinton." The view that heart disease is a manifestation of a character defect finds favour with some people. It can be politically convenient to blame the sick for their own misfortune. It lessens governments' obligations to care for them.

> *The view that heart disease is a manifestation of a character defect finds favour with some people.*

SO IT MUST BE GENETIC

Doctors see many patients with heart disease who have healthy lifestyles. Our usual response is to say it must be genetic. Bill Clinton blamed his genes. There was a history of heart disease in his mother's family. "It must be genetic" is a comfortable view. The patient is freed from blame; and the doctor no longer has to engage with the issue. It is fate decreed by the tyranny of genes. No one knows which particular genes they are, despite a huge investment that has deformed medical research and deprived other areas with more immediate prospects of improving health. The hope is that with more time, and even more money, things will work out. Yet within only a hundred years a once rare disease has become the most common cause of death in the world. Genes do not change so rapidly. It takes thousands of years. Furthermore genes are not automatic switches: they have to be turned-on.

> *...within only a hundred years a once rare disease has become the most common cause of death in the world. Genes do not change so rapidly.*

Whether they are is conditioned by what is happening to other parts and functions within an individual. Our genetic inheritance from our parents is not a Stalinist dictatorship within our bodies, able to command chronic disease and premature death. Genes are

Genes are part of a democracy, and what they do in one person they may not do in another.

part of a democracy, and what they do in one person they may not do in another.

The long and fruitless search for the causes of coronary heart disease contrasts sharply with the progress made with its treatment. There is constant pressure on doctors to improve treatment, but little pressure to prevent disease. This is surprising since, while patients are grateful for better treatments, they would prefer not to be ill in the first place. A Chinese physician wrote that inferior doctors treat the sick while mediocre doctors diagnose illness before it becomes apparent; but superior doctors prevent illness. For us inferior doctors who seek to become superior ones there is a powerful clue.

...while patients are grateful for better treatments, they would prefer not to be ill in the first place.

SUMMARY

Attempts to prevent coronary heart disease have largely failed. The disease was rare one hundred years ago; but now it is the most common cause of death in the world. High dietary fat, low fiber, high salt, high sugar, too much meat have all been suspected to cause it. Yet none of them, nor any other aspect of lifestyle such as smoking, goes more than a small way to explaining why one person has heart disease while another does not. When President Clinton was found to have heart disease he was told that it was due to his eating too much pizza, and to faulty, though as yet undiscovered, genes. When, in large trials, people have improved their lifestyles the reduction in heart disease has been very small. A new way forward is needed.

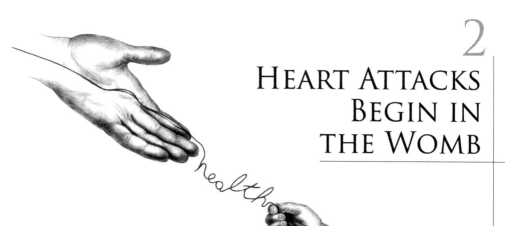

HEART ATTACKS BEGIN IN THE WOMB

WHY DO POOR PEOPLE GET MORE HEART DISEASE?

Across the US heart disease is commoner in states in the Southeast and Southwest. The highest levels are in West Virginia, where 10 percent of adults have the disease, followed by Kentucky, where 9 percent have it. The lowest level, 5 percent, is in Colorado. Within any state poorer people are more at risk than wealthier people. Those who are poorly educated are more at risk than the well educated: one in ten people who did not finish high school have the disease compared to one in twenty college graduates. This is surprising. Heart disease increased rapidly as the US became wealthier and better educated. Why then has the disease settled among the poor? In Europe there is the same link with poverty.

> Heart disease increased rapidly as the US became wealthier and better educated. Why then has the disease settled among the poor?

The large variations in heart disease within the US are unexplained. "The explanation would come from differences in cultural norms, poverty rates and other social factors, and not environmental causes" wrote the New York Times (February 16, 2007), rehearsing a spurious and obsolete orthodoxy. Put another way "the people of West Virginia and Kentucky are responsible for their own misfortunes. They drop out of high school, sit around, gorge, get fat, smoke and so, inevitably, their lives are brought to a premature and self-inflicted end".

A study published more than twenty years ago, and ignored, showed that differences between states in their rates of coronary heart disease were predicted by past differences in the numbers of infants who died from diarrhea. In the past large numbers of babies died from diarrhea, which was common in poor families whose homes lacked sanitation. The higher the infant death rates fifty or so years ago, the higher the levels of heart disease today. This was a clue that heart disease might be linked to poor living conditions in childhood. It was, however, impossible to follow up this lead because many American people move from one place to another through their lives. Their heart attacks occur far from where they were born, and there is no record of their early health and growth or of the conditions they lived in as children. European populations are less mobile, and in some countries there are records of children's health and growth that go back many years. Ideas about the early origins of heart disease have been developed through studies that use these European records.

In Britain, as in the US, deaths from heart disease are commoner in poor areas; in the northern towns which became the focus of the industrial revolution in the nineteenth century, and whose dreadful social conditions attracted the attention of Karl Marx; and in the poor farmlands in the west whose fertile soil was scoured off as the glaciers melted eastwards at the end of the last Ice Age. The disparity in death rates from heart disease across Britain, and hence the disparity in life expectancy, is a large one. If each area of Britain had the low rates of heart disease which prevail in the fertile farmlands in the east, the rich lands which once enticed Viking marauders to cross the seas in tiny boats, the increase in life expectancy would be greater than would be achieved by the immediate abolition of all forms of cancer!

Today people in the poor areas have similar lifestyles to people elsewhere. They eat the same food; they have similar levels of overweight and obesity, and similar smoking habits. They live in places that are historically poor, but their lives today are little different to those of other people. A government committee set up to examine their poor health shrugged its shoulders and concluded that "much, we feel, can only be understood in terms of the more diffuse consequences of the class structure," a meaningless statement which echoed the 'miasma' theory for malaria. Before its transmission by mosquitoes was discovered, the disease was attributed to the miasma, or bad air, of marshlands. Malaria literally means bad air. "Diffuse consequences of the class structure" suggested that committee knew that the British class system was the murderer responsible for all these deaths, but they had not been able to figure out the murder weapon.

THE TWO WORLDS

If it is not their lifestyles and behaviours which make poor people get more heart disease, could it be that they are more vulnerable to harmful influences to which everyone is exposed. Inevitably, thoughts about vulnerability lead to genes. But the idea that poorer people are made vulnerable to heart disease through their genes is untenable. The people who flocked to work in the factories of the industrial revolution, or settled in the farmlands of Kentucky, came from many parts of the country, and from other countries around the world. Why should their descendants have a unique genetic make-up that gives them heart disease? The argument that poor

The argument that poor people, from inferior stock, are genetically disadvantaged, has a tarnished history...

Our constitution is much more than our genetic inheritance.

people, from inferior stock, are genetically disadvantaged, has a tarnished history which is discussed in Chapter 9. We are all familiar with the idea that some people are constitutionally vulnerable to disease: I am indifferent to the pollen count on a summer's day, but it profoundly changes the well-being of my son, who gets asthma. Our constitution is much more than our genetic inheritance.

Early thoughts on the vulnerability of poorer people to heart disease came from a Norwegian family doctor, Anders Forsdahl. In the long winter evenings of northern Norway he pondered why people living above the Arctic Circle had death rates that were 25% higher than those in other parts of Norway. The weather was worse, but social and economic conditions were similar to those elsewhere. Immigrants from Finland had the highest rates. Their lifestyles were similar to those of their neighbors but in the past, like many immigrant communities in the US, they had been short of food and had lived in poor, overcrowded homes. He concluded that poor living conditions in childhood predisposed men and women to heart disease. He did not pursue these ideas further, but he carried ideas about the origins of heart disease back from the western lifestyles of adults to the poor living conditions of children. As it turned out one more step back was required, from children to babies in the womb.

In the womb a baby grows through the division of its cells. Beginning as one cell the fertilized egg passes through 42 cycles of cell division as it changes from egg, to embryo, to baby. After birth only a further five cycles of division are needed to change the infant into an adult.

Our constitution is largely wrought during life in the womb.

Most of the organs and systems of the human body are complete at birth. Key organs like the heart and the kidney, important tissues such as muscle, are almost fully formed. After birth they merely enlarge. Our constitution is largely wrought during life in the womb. The poet William Blake wrote, "Man brings all that he has or can have into the world with him. Man is born like a garden ready planted and sown".

The first clue that heart disease begins during life in the womb came from London, which has exceptionally low rates of heart disease. Yet historically much of London, the London described by Charles Dickens, was poor. I have a photograph, taken a hundred years ago, of children in a London slum waiting for free food. They are thin, dirty and barefoot. One boy has shoes but his toes are sticking out above the soles. Why did such children have low rates of heart disease when they grew up?

In our lives we live in two worlds, the world within our mothers, where we are wrought, and the world into which we are born, where we become independent. In those days London babies began life in a kind world, within well-nourished mothers, but they left that world for an unkind one. They were born into crowded, unsanitary homes, where they were at risk of diarrhea, bronchitis, pneumonia and measles. Large numbers of them died in the months after birth. During the First World War the Bishop of London wrote, "While nine soldiers died every hour in 1915, twelve babies died every hour, so that it was more dangerous to be a baby than a soldier." Writing of the London poor, Charles Booth, who mapped the social conditions of every street in London in 1889, recorded that

> In our lives we live in two worlds, the world within our mothers, where we are wrought, and the world into which we are born, where we become independent.

"their life is the life of savages with vicissitudes of extreme hardship and occasional excess. Their food is of the coarsest description, and their only luxury is drink". In this harsh world babies thrived in the womb and few were born dead. How could this be?

The answer is that many of the mothers were not themselves born in London, but grew up in the fertile farmlands of southern and eastern England. Food was plentiful, but wages were low. As teenage girls, they were attracted to London by the high wages paid to domestic servants. Booth wrote that they were "mainly the cream of the youth of the villages travelling not so often vaguely in search of work as definitely to seek a known economic advantage." In London they lived in the homes of the rich and shared the same food. When they married and became pregnant, they were well-nourished. Their babies flourished in the womb and at birth were healthy and well grown. In later life these babies had low rates of heart disease.

SUMMARY

Across the US, and in Europe, poorer people have the highest rates of heart disease. One in ten people who did not finish high school have the disease compared to one in twenty college graduates. The disease is also more common in historically poorer states such as West Virginia and Kentucky. In the last century the disease increased rapidly as the US became wealthier and better educated. Why then has it settled among the poor? No aspect of the lifestyles of the poor can explain this. An alternative explanation is that poorer people are more vulnerable to damaging components of a western lifestyle shared by rich and poor alike. New research now suggests that poor people are made vulnerable to heart disease through the conditions they experience in the womb.

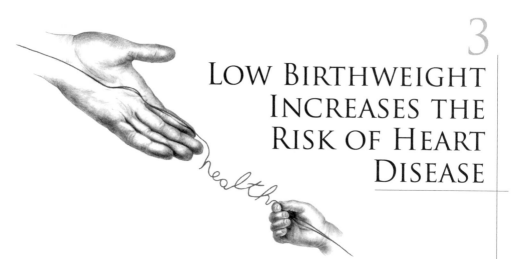

3

LOW BIRTHWEIGHT INCREASES THE RISK OF HEART DISEASE

IN POOR CONDITIONS, with lack of food, or stress or other hardships, living things grow more slowly. Babies are no exception. If a mother is badly nourished, or ill, or for other reasons unable to supply food to her baby, the baby will grow more slowly and have a lower birthweight than a baby in favourable conditions. If the low rates of heart disease in Londoners reflect their good experiences in the womb then the disease should be less common among people who had a high birthweight.

> *In poor conditions, with lack of food, or stress or other hardships, living things grow more slowly. Babies are no exception.*

To test this idea has required studies of a kind never undertaken before. Large groups of babies born 50 or more years ago, whose birthweights were recorded, have had to be traced through their lives to see which of them have died and what they died of. Such studies were more readily carried out in Europe than in the USA. In some European countries people have a unique identification number, which allows research workers to trace them through their lifetimes. The first of these studies was carried out in Britain.

In the early years of the twentieth century, there was concern about the physical deterioration of the British nation. In 1902 reports in the national press claimed that up to two thirds of the young men who volunteered to join the army had to be rejected because they were not fit. A government committee set up in the following year drew a shocking picture of the nation's children—malnourished, poorly housed, deprived. Worse still the birth rate was declining. There was talk of national decline, and the doom of western civilization.

The challenge was to improve the nutrition and health of mothers and their children. Responding to this a young nurse in the county of Hertfordshire set up an "army" of trained nurses to attend women in childbirth and to advise mothers on how to keep their infants and children healthy after birth. From that time onwards when any woman in the county had a baby she was attended by a midwife. The midwife recorded the birthweight and a nurse visited the baby's home repeatedly throughout the first year after birth to advise the mother. When the infant was one year old she weighed it again. The details of each visit were written down in ledgers, and these have survived to the present day.

In the first study 15,000 men and women born in the county before 1930 were traced. 3,000 of them were already dead, almost half of them from heart disease. A disproportionate number of these deaths had occurred among people who had had low birthweights. People who weighed 10 pounds or more at birth had half the rate of fatal heart attacks as occurred among people who weighed 5 pounds or less. It was not that 5 pound babies had high death rates and everyone who weighed more than that had similar, lower rates. Rather there was a progressive fall in death rates from heart disease across the range of birthweights. Fewer people who were 7-pound

Fewer people who were 7-pound babies had heart disease than people who were 6-pound babies: those who were 9-pound babies were at lower risk than those who weighed 8 pounds.

babies had heart disease than people who were 6-pound babies: those who were 9-pound babies were at lower risk than those who weighed 8 pounds. Studies in the US, in other European countries and in India have confirmed this initial finding, and have also shown that it is not babies who were small because they were born prematurely who are at increased risk of later heart disease, but babies who were small because they grew slowly.

People sometimes ask, "I only weighed five pounds when I was born, but I was a twin: do I have a problem?" To which the answer is "not necessarily." A baby that weighs five pounds because it had to share the womb with another human being is biologically different from a single-born baby of the same weight. Some twins seem to settle for less at an early stage of pregnancy and grow slowly. Others grow more rapidly but in late pregnancy, when the babies are large and the competition for food severe, they are unable to sustain their growth. The consequences of these two paths of growth will be different, though as yet little is known about this.

The early studies in Hertfordshire showed that babies who did not thrive after birth and gained weight slowly while they were breast fed and weaned, also had a higher risk of heart attacks in later life. Men who weighed 18 pounds or less at one year of age were three times more likely to have a fatal heart attack than men who weighed 27 pounds or more. Even among the men whose birthweights were above the average of 8 pounds slow weight gain during infancy doubled the risk of heart attacks. Few studies have been able to develop these early observations because, unlike birthweights, which were often recorded in the past, records of the growth of infants are scarce.

…that babies who did not thrive after birth and gained weight slowly while they were breast fed and weaned, also had a higher risk of heart attacks in later life.

There is, however, one remarkable set of records, in Helsinki, Finland. In the first part of the last century Finland had exceptionally high rates of infant and child death. Around one in five children died. To counter this child welfare clinics were established. They were free and all mothers were encouraged to bring their children to them regularly. At each visit the children were weighed, their height were measured, and notes were written about their illnesses and living conditions. Records of all this activity were kept at the clinics and later, when the children had grown up, they were transferred to the city archives. And there they remained, undisturbed, unused, until fifteen years ago when Finnish researchers studying the early origins of heart disease and diabetes discovered them. An early finding from what is known as "Helsinki birth cohort" was confirmation that slow weight gain from birth to two years of age increased the risk of later heart disease, just as was found in Hertfordshire.

When published the findings in Hertfordshire met with disbelief. How could the weights of babies and infants recorded long ago in cottages, huts and hovels, measured by the light of candles and lanterns with the simplest of weighing scales, predict heart disease fifty years later? All that these findings showed, the critics argued fiercely, was that little babies were born into different kinds of homes than big babies, poorer homes with worse educated parents; and as a result they grew up to have worse, less 'healthy' lifestyles. It was these lifestyles that led to their high rates of heart disease, not their experiences in the womb. For some medical scientists, the self-appointed gurus who preached about adult lifestyles, their way of life seemed to be under threat. They walked out of medical meetings in protest, and complained in the medical press. But more studies were done and the evidence grew. Among 100,000 nurses studied in the US those with lower birthweights had more heart disease irrespective of their lifestyles and living conditions.

Among 100,000 nurses studied in the US those with lower birthweights had more heart disease irrespective of their lifestyles and living conditions.

PEOPLE BORN WITH DIFFERENT WEIGHTS ARE DIFFERENT FOR LIFE

4-pound babies are ten times more likely to die in the weeks after birth than 9-pound ones. They die because their struggle to grow in the womb has left them unable to adjust to the new and dangerous world into which they are born. Within minutes of birth a baby casts off its single life-line, the placenta, and must rapidly establish others. Breast milk must be absorbed through the untested digestive system; air absorbed through the lungs; and the kidneys must begin to clear the body's waste. Bigger babies are fitter, better able to achieve these internal changes by which their lives are preserved.

But why should small babies continue to be at less fit, long after the transition from the womb to the outside world has been accomplished? One answer is that their bodies do not function as well. We bring into the world all the kidney cells we will ever have, and most of the muscle cells. Small babies have fewer cells. As we age we lose cells, and for people who were small at birth functional ability may become critical. Their kidneys may no longer be able to maintain blood pressure at normal levels, and their muscles may become too weak to sustain activity. It is, however, more complex than that. The organs of the body do not act alone, anymore than do the machines in a factory. They act in concert, as systems. The flow of blood depends on the coordinated activity of the heart, arteries and kidneys. Coordination requires signalling, by hormones and nerves.

Coordinated by the brain, the body's systems maintain an inner constancy despite an ever-changing world outside. We each have a unique "internal environment" which conditions our responses to the external environment. When the fire alarm rings some

> *Health depends on the ability to maintain a constant internal environment in the face of challenges from the outside world. People who were small at birth seem less able to do this.*

people do one thing, some another. When excess food is consumed some peoples' bodies burn it off while others store it and become fat. The internal environment is established during development in the womb; thereafter it is relatively constant. Health depends on the ability to maintain a constant internal environment in the face of challenges from the outside world. People who were small at birth seem less able to do this. This makes them more vulnerable to disease.

SUMMARY

In adverse conditions due to lack of food, stress or other hardships, living things grow more slowly. Babies are no exception. Studies around the world have now shown that people who had low birthweight are at higher risk of heart disease. People who weighed 7-pounds are at lower risk than those who weighed 6-pounds: 9-pound babies are at lower risk than 8 pound ones. The people at risk are those who were small at birth because they grew slowly, rather than because they were born prematurely. Low weight gain in the first two years after birth also increases the risk of later heart disease.

Health depends on the ability to maintain an internal constancy in the face of challenges from the outside world. People who were small at birth and during infancy are less able to do this and it makes them more vulnerable to heart disease.

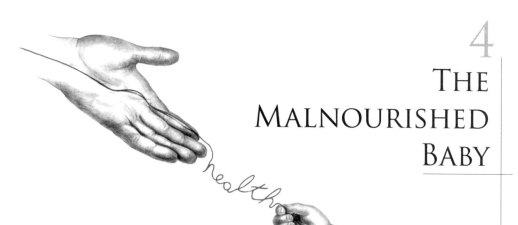

4

THE
MALNOURISHED
BABY

BABIES ARE PLASTIC

Children in America today are taller and reach puberty earlier than their parents did. This is clearly not the result of genetic change, because it has occurred too rapidly. It is a speeding up of growth and development in response to a better environment. It is a simple demonstration that human beings, like all living things, are 'plastic'. As we develop in the womb and after birth our organs are pliable, moulded by the environment, by the food we get, by adversity and stress. These determine how fast we grow, how rapidly we develop and the quality of our systems and structures.

Within the broad limits imposed by our genes, each of us had a range of options for our lives. Our environment in the womb and in the months after birth selected the particular path of growth and development we followed. Human development has been likened to cooking. The genes we acquire at conception are a general recipe for making a human being. They specify

Within the broad limits imposed by our genes, each of us had a range of options for our lives. Our environment in the womb and in the months after birth selected the particular path of growth and development we followed.

23

our sex, and traits such as the colour of our skin and eyes, but the unique human being that we each became is the product of the general recipe, and the specific ingredients and biological signals we received from our mothers. Look around a nursery of newborn babies. See the fat one, the thin one, the short one, the one with the large head. Each baby would have had a different size and shape had its experiences in the womb been different.

The common lizard is a successful creature that inhabits much of the earth. Its success is due to its plasticity. In different places it grows and matures at different rates. In France the lizards living in the southern mountains grow more slowly than those living in the meadows of Brittany, where it is warmer and food is plentiful. They do not become sexually mature until they are two years old, while those in Brittany become mature at one. If, after hatching, young lizards from both places are raised in a laboratory in Paris, their lives are identical. The faster growth and earlier puberty of Americans and Europeans today is as though, like the lizard, we have moved ourselves from the austerity of the mountains to the plenty of the meadows.

The genes acquired at conception are known as the 'genotype'. They are capable of producing a range of body sizes and shapes and differences in structure and function within the body. These are referred to as 'phenotypes'.

The genes acquired at conception are known as the 'genotype'. They are capable of producing a range of body sizes and shapes and differences in structure and function within the body. These different bodies are referred to as 'phenotypes'. It is our final phenotype that governs our lives. When a man is fleeing from a charging bull, neither the bull nor anyone else is interested in his genotype. The issue is how fast and how far he can run. This is his phenotype.

Darwin first described how evolution occurs over many generations through natural selection of genes. Natural selection chooses animals that can avoid predators and survive and who are attractive to the opposite sex. Darwin was also aware that the environment produces variation within one generation. "When a variation is of the slightest use to a being," he wrote, "we cannot tell how much of it to attribute to the accumulative action of natural selection, and how much to the conditions of life. Thus, it is well known to furriers that animals of the same species have thicker and better fur the more severe the climate is under which they have lived; but who can tell how much of this difference may be due to the warmest-clad individuals having been favoured and preserved during many generations, and how much to the direct action of the severe climate". Among young domestic animals, he noted, cold weather stimulated the growth of hair.

Developmental plasticity enables the production of phenotypes that are better suited to their surroundings than would be possible if the same phenotype was produced regardless of the environment. It affects our life history, our lifespan and the way our body works. The development of the sweat glands illustrates plasticity in humans. In the last century Japanese military expansion took their soldiers and settlers into unfamiliar climates. There were wide differences in Japanese people's abilities to adapt to hot climates. Physiologists were told to study this and found that it was related to the number of functioning sweat glands. Each of us has a different density of functioning sweat glands on our skin. Some of us have many glands, sweat freely and adapt well to hot weather; others have fewer glands and suffer in warm weather. It must be genetic, would be the fashionable response today, but the Japanese looked more deeply and made an interesting discovery.

> *Developmental plasticity enables the production of phenotypes that are better suited to their surroundings than would be possible if the same phenotype was produced regardless of the environment.*

At birth, the sweat glands are in place but they are inactive. In the next three years a proportion of them begin to function. In hot countries many become functional, in cold countries only a few. After three years the number that is active is fixed. Glands that are inactive remain so forever. The story of the sweat gland illustrates a simple but important phenomenon. Many of the body's systems need to be stimulated by the environment before they function and assume their final form. The development of the sweat glands is triggered by heat. It is neither good nor bad to have few working sweat glands. It is merely appropriate to life in colder places. If in later life the environment changes, it may be a disadvantage. Japanese soldiers who grew up in colder parts of the country struggled when they were sent to the tropics. For the sweat gland it is the environment after birth that determines its destiny. For much of the body, however, it is the environment before birth.

SENSITIVE PERIODS IN A BABY'S DEVELOPMENT

During 'sensitive' or 'critical' periods adverse conditions, such as undernutrition, will change a tissue or system permanently.

For the sweat glands, like many different tissues and systems of the body, there is a critical period of development during which they are plastic and sensitive to the environment. After that plasticity is lost and functional ability becomes fixed. During 'sensitive' or 'critical' periods adverse conditions, such as undernutrition, will change a tissue or system permanently. When the sensitive period is over the effects of under nutrition have become 'hard-wired' in the body, preserved for a lifetime. The timing of these sensitive periods differs for different organs. The kidney, for example, has a sensitive period around the thirty-fourth week of pregnancy, at a time when its cells are dividing rapidly. The sensitive period for muscle is earlier. For most organs and tissues the sensitive period occurs before birth, although our knowledge

For most organs and tissues the sensitive period occurs before birth...

of their precise timing is incomplete. The sweat glands are an exception to this.

Experiments on rats have provided a striking illustration of sensitive periods. When a female rat was given an injection of the male hormone, testosterone, on the fifth day after birth her sexual characteristics developed normally, but she never mated. One injection had irreversibly altered the release of the hormones which drove her sexuality. If, however, the same injection of testosterone was given when the animal was 20 days old, it had no effect. Thus there is a critical, sensitive period in which the animal's sexual physiology is plastic and can be permanently changed. After that period plasticity is lost.

SETTING ITS RATE OF GROWTH

The baby establishes its rate of growth soon after it is conceived, and tries to maintain this rate throughout its time in the womb. After birth, the infant resets the trajectory and sets off with a new growth tempo. The rate of growth that is established in early pregnancy is important because it determines the baby's demand for food in later gestation, when its food requirements are greatest. A baby that is large at any point in time needs more food, and so does a baby that is growing fast. If a baby is not adequately nourished, it is more likely to have to slow its growth if it is growing rapidly.

If a baby in the womb becomes undernourished, its immediate response is to use its own stores of food for the energy it needs to continue to grow. If it continues to be undernourished, its rate of growth will slow. If nutrition is restored after a few days, the baby resumes growth at the previous rate, but prolonged undernutrition may slow growth irreversibly. A baby's ability to slow its growth when under nourished may be useful, 'adaptive', because it reduces the amount of energy it needs. We use the word 'adaptive' to describe the changes by which living things overcome the challenges of life. People sometimes talk about growth and development as though they are unalterable consequences of genes. "John is intelligent and growing tall just like his father." True perhaps, but John may not have become so intelligent in less stimulating surroundings,

People talk about children growing to their "genetic potential", when the reality is that children grow according to their circumstances.

and his growth will slow if he is undernourished, ill or stressed in other ways. People talk about children growing to their "genetic potential", when the reality is that children grow according to their circumstances. The weeds in your backyard are of different heights, not simply because they are from different types of plant but because of differences in sunshine, moisture and nutrients. Development and growth are not like musical symphonies, commanded by a single set of detailed instructions; they are like jazz, dynamic processes with improvisations and elaborations that depend on circumstances.

Development and growth are not like musical symphonies, commanded by a single set of detailed instructions; they are like jazz, dynamic processes with improvisations and elaborations that depend on circumstances.

Whether an animal's responses to adversity during development are adaptive, helping it to survive, or simply the result of the constraints imposed on it are recurring themes. Biologists have always been fascinated by the way animals cope with life in a temporary pond: shrimps, tadpoles, beetles, larvae, packed into a space smaller than your living room. One day it dries up. Some of the creatures die, and the species has to recolonize it again when it refills. Others lay eggs in the mud or burrow into it themselves and wait for the pond to refill. The tadpoles speed up their development, grow legs and hop away as frogs. Is this a clever trick that allows the tadpoles to survive? Or is it simply a mechanical response to less food or warmer water?

BOYS ARE MORE VULNERABLE THAN GIRLS

In the US and Europe, heart disease is more common among men. Those who subscribe to the view that heart disease is primarily the result of lifestyle explain this by the more reckless, cavalier lifestyles of men, and their predisposition to smoke, drink and overeat. It used to be thought that women were also protected from heart disease by their estrogens, but this now seems unlikely. If heart disease originates during development, why should men be more vulnerable than women?

Shortage of food during development may not affect the two sexes equally. The faster growing sex, the boy in humans, is more vulnerable. In humans and other mammals, and among those birds in which the two sexes have different body size, males grow faster and for longer than females and need more food. Among sheep, young rams eat 15% more food than ewes of the same age. In the nest, young male blackbirds eat 30% more food than young females. Males are more vulnerable when food is scarce. Generally, in mammals, if mothers are in poor condition their male offspring are more severely affected. In humans, more sons than daughters die in the womb and during childhood. The advantage of large body size when males compete with each other to reproduce is offset by the greater risk of death when food is short. When soldiers fight hand-to-hand tall, strong men are favored. When captured and poorly fed the tall soldiers die first, because they need more food.

The reproductive success of males is more variable than that of females. Some males have many partners, many children; others have none. The success of a young male may be more readily jeopardized by poor conditions than the success of a female. Among red deer on the island of Rum, Scotland, males with low birth weight have fewer offspring, but this does not apply to females with low birth weight. The Hertfordshire men who were small at birth were less likely to marry: around 20 per cent of men who weighed 5½ pounds or less at birth remained unmarried in middle age compared with only 5 percent of men who weighed 8 pounds or more. This was not simply the result of men who were larger at birth being taller as adults and hence more attractive to women. At any given height, those who were smaller at birth were less likely to marry. It seems that if a baby boy's growth is restricted before birth some aspect of partner selection is changed. Whether it is sexuality, socialization, personality or emotional responses is not known.

It is folk-lore that strong, dominant women tend to produce sons. Among animals it is a better option for a mother in good condition to invest in sons because, on average, they will produce more children than daughters. If the lives of sheep, blackbirds, red deer seem to you interesting but remote from the human experience, consider this. In the famine in Holland during the Second World War the proportion of boys born fell sharply: boys were more vulnerable to undernutrition. In Britain during the First World War, while young men died in their thousands in the trenches, the proportion of boys being born increased. How did this work? A recent theory proposes that periods of intense and repeated sexual intercourse, as might occur when a soldier returned home on leave, are more likely to favor male sperm reaching the egg. Male sperm swim faster than female sperm, but female sperm survive for longer. The processes through which the proportion of boys born varies from year to year are not understood, but these fluctuations make the point that human reproduction is governed by laws that govern other animals. The human mother provides the arena for biological processes we little understand, and once they have begun we have little control over them.

TRADING OFF ONE PART OF THE BODY AGAINST ANOTHER

A baby receiving an inadequate supply of food or oxygen may protect its brain by diverting more blood to it. On any day of the week, in the ultrasound rooms of maternity hospitals, babies may be seen to have sacrificed the growth of one part of their body for the benefit of another. They can do this because they have three junctions in their circulation through which blood may be diverted to one organ and away from another. These junctions close after birth. The human brain is large and protecting it in times of scarcity

> On any day of the week, in the ultrasound rooms of maternity hospitals, babies may be seen to have sacrificed the growth of one part of their body for the benefit of another.

has exaggerated costs for other parts of the body, notably the liver which is large in a baby, but also for other organs such as the lung and the kidney and for muscle. Protecting these is not an immediate priority as, until birth, the mother performs many of their functions on the baby's behalf. We are beginning to understand how 'trading-off' can permanently change an organ's function and lead to disease in later life.

Trading off is a universal experience which humans share with other living things, because during development there is usually insufficient food available to perfect every structure and every function of the body. An "ideal" creature would reproduce immediately after birth, produce large numbers of large offspring and repeat this through a long lifespan. It would also out-number its competitors, escape from its predators and catch its own prey easily. This is not possible. The needs of one activity conflict with those of another. The activities

> Trading off is a universal experience which humans share with other living things, because during development there is usually insufficient food available to perfect every structure and every function of the body.

required to avoid predators differ from those which catch prey.

There must be trade-offs in which the benefits of increasing one activity are set against its disadvantages.

The life of the Caddis fly is an interesting example. The eggs hatch into larvae which live and feed in fresh water. Thereafter, while they change into pupae and then to adult flies, they do not feed, and must live off their food stores, the food 'capital' acquired by the larvae. The fly's body has two main parts, an abdomen which consists almost entirely of the reproductive system, and a chest which contains the wings. While it is a pupa food from the stores is allocated to each part, after which the final shape of the body is fixed. If food is scarce because the stores are small, to which body part should it be allocated? Should reproduction be favored over flight, or vice versa?

The answer, like that to many questions in biology, is that it depends on the circumstances. One species of caddis fly larva is a scavenger living in streams. The eggs hatch in the autumn, and a long 10-month period of larval development through winter and spring is followed by a brief adult life in the summer. Adults emerge from the pupae, mate and die within only a few days. In contrast, another species of caddis fly eats vegetation, and lives in temporary ponds that dry up in summer. It has a shorter period of larval life than the stream dweller. It has, however, a much longer adult life, that lasts for 4 months, as it has to survive until the ponds re-fill in the fall.

In both these species, when larvae are under nourished the adults are smaller. The adult stream-dwellers, however, preserve their abdomens and hence the capacity to reproduce, at the expense of their chests and their capacity to fly. The pond-dwellers do the reverse. Preserving the ability to fly is unimportant to the stream-dweller for whom the imperative is to reproduce in the few hectic hours of its adult life. The pond-dweller, however, has to survive through the summer until winter rains replenish the ponds in which it breeds.

The lizards in Brittany grow faster, and reproduce earlier, than those in the southern mountains of France, but they live shorter lives. They trade off lifespan against the advantages of rapid growth and early reproduction. Reproducing at an earlier age is a biological gain, because it reduces the likelihood of death before reproduction and thereby increases the likelihood of passing genes to the next generation. For the lizards in the mountains rapid growth is not an option, because there is insufficient food; but they are able to invest in the development of processes which will maintain and repair their bodies and prolong their lives.

Poor food, competition, bad weather and predators are some of the reasons why humans and other animals face food shortages during development. They may be born late in the breeding season, when worsening conditions reduce food supply; or their parents may fail to make adequate provision for them. Animals that give birth to their young in eggs have a 'capital' strategy for development. The food in the egg is the capital and the young have no daily additional 'income'. Reptiles and many birds hatch from their eggs with their bodies close to their final form. They are therefore more vulnerable to lack of nutritional 'capital' than insects, which are hatched as larvae and have opportunities to compensate for lack of capital before they reach their adult form. A butterfly lays its eggs on the lushest vegetation so that the caterpillars will have the best start in life.

The human baby lives off income. This differs widely between babies, even between the babies of one mother. Mothers wonder why their babies can be so different to each other. Partly this is because the babies' source of income, the mother's body and diet, changes between pregnancies; but it also reflects differences in the supply lines to the baby. Embryos can implant in many different parts of the mothers womb. Not all parts are equally good, just as seeds grow better in one parts of a garden than another. Unlike the butterfly the mother cannot choose the spot.

Embryos can implant in many different parts of the mothers womb. Not all parts are equally good...

Variations in a Baby's Food Supply

Through their lives people who weighed eight pounds at birth experience less heart disease, stroke, high blood pressure and diabetes than people who weighed seven pounds. People who weighed seven pounds have less than those who weighed six pounds. This is surprising. Most people, most doctors, would have expected that while someone who was small at birth, say 5 pounds or less, might not be as healthy as everyone else, whether a person was seven, eight or nine pounds would be of no consequence. This is not the case and the implications are profound. The growth of a baby depends ultimately on the food it receives. Therefore what were once regarded as normal variations in the food supply from healthy mothers to normal healthy babies are now known to have important life-long effects.

...what were once regarded as normal variations in the food supply from healthy mothers to normal healthy babies are now known to have important life-long effects.

Through this book "people with low birthweight" is shorthand for "people born at full term whose birthweights were towards the lower end of the scale of normality, which ranges from 5 pounds or less up to 10 or more".

Underlying the graded relation between birthweight and later health there may be a gradation in the level of trade-offs babies had to make in the womb. Less food leads to more trading off, and to smaller babies. More trading off could involve graded increases in the sacrifice of particular organs or systems. There could also be switches, whereby a trade off either happens or it does not.

Darwin was impressed by the extraordinary variation in the shape and size of the horns of male beetles. Within the same species the horns range can from a tiny knob to structures longer than the entire body. Darwin thought they were mere ornaments, whose purpose was to attract females; but we now know that they are weapons, used when males fight each other to gain access to females. The largest beetles, those who were the best nourished as larvae, have the longest horns. Are long horns simply an extravagance open only to the better-nourished animals? It seems that they are. Experiments show that increasing amounts of food do not result in progressively longer and longer horns. Rather there is a threshold of feeding below which the beetle has no horns and above which it has fully developed horns, whose size is dependent on the beetles' body size. A threshold implies the existence of a switch, turned on once a certain feeding level is reached. Whether human babies have switches of this kind remains largely unknown.

BABIES WITH DIFFERENT SHAPES

It is simple and convenient to weigh a baby. But weight is a crude measure of the size of a body. It may be adequate for a newly caught fish, but not for a newly born baby. Different paths of growth, rapid growth followed by slow growth, sustained moderate growth, can produce babies with the same birthweights. Birthweight tells us nothing about the growth of different parts of the body. In the past midwives measured babies lengths, from the top of their heads to their feet. They measured the circumferences of their heads, their arms, chests and abdomens. Many thousands of people alive today had such measurements recorded. They could be used to make drawings of how they looked

Birthweight tells us nothing about the growth of different parts of the body.

at birth, drawings that would be recognised by their mothers. The drawings would also give an insight into the trade offs they made in the womb. A newborn baby with a large head in relation to its body has maintained brain growth, which begins early in pregnancy, but has been unable to sustain growth of its trunk later on. A thin baby has failed to make enough muscle during the 'critical' period for muscle growth in late pregnancy, or has been unable to accumulate fat.

If a baby is undernourished throughout pregnancy it will be small but proportional at birth, a miniature. Many Chinese babies are like this. If undernutrition begins in mid or late pregnancy the baby will be thin or short. Many Indian babies are born like this. The World Health Organisation compared newborn babies in China, India and Sweden. The Chinese babies had an average weight of more than 7 pounds, but they had smaller heads and shorter bodies than the Indian babies, who weighed only 6½ pounds because they were thin. The Swedish babies weighed more than 8 pounds, and had the largest heads and the longest bodies. The Chinese babies, although the least successful in terms of brain and body growth, were fatter than the Swedish babies. In this way birthweight conceals important differences between babies.

Though they may have the same birthweights, babies that have small bodies in relation to the size of their heads, babies that are thin or short, have each followed different paths of growth. The size of their organs will be different; and their bodies will function differently. Thin or stunted newborn babies are not a thing of the past. Many newborn Americans are thin or short. Why do they get more chronic disease in later life?

Thin or stunted newborn babies are not a thing of the past. Many newborn Americans are thin or short.

SUMMARY

Like all living things as they develop babies are molded by the food they receive. This determines how fast they grow and the quality of the systems and structures they develop. During what are called "sensitive periods" of development malnutrition changes a tissue or system permanently. When the sensitive period is over the effects of malnutrition will have become "hard-wired" in the body, preserved for a lifetime. For most organs and tissues the sensitive period occurs before birth.

A baby protects the growth of its brain at the expense of other parts of the body, such as the lung and kidney. Protecting these is not an immediate priority as, until birth, the mother performs many of their functions on the baby's behalf. These organs are 'traded off'. We are beginning to understand how 'trading-off' can permanently change an organ's function and lead to disease in later life.

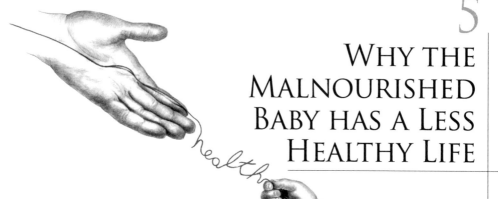

5
WHY THE MALNOURISHED BABY HAS A LESS HEALTHY LIFE

THAT WONDERFUL ORGAN

Evolution has produced a number of solutions to the problem of how best to attach babies to their mothers. While the placentas of pigs and sheep have four layers of cells separating the blood streams of mother and baby, the human placenta has only two. Because of this intimate contact food passes more readily from the mother to the baby. This allows the human brain, which requires much of the food, to develop to an advanced state before birth. The placenta has three main functions: it is the gate through which food and oxygen are transferred from the mother; it is a factory that makes hormones for both mother and baby; and it is a barrier that protects the baby from the mother's immune system, which could otherwise reject the baby as 'foreign' to her body.

The placenta has three main functions: it is the gate through which food and oxygen are transferred from the mother; it is a factory that makes hormones for both mother and baby; and it is a barrier that protects the baby from the mother's immune system…

If a pregnant woman is badly nourished the placenta may not be able to develop fully. This has been a source of concern for a long while.

> *If a pregnant woman is badly nourished the placenta may not be able to develop fully.*

In 1884, the Encyclopaedia Britannica, commenting on the poor living conditions of women working in factories, stated that "the building of the placenta by the mother and the performance of the function of that wonderful organ requires certain favoring conditions. These are certainly not to be found in factory labor."

In mid-pregnancy the placenta grows faster than the baby; thereafter it grows more slowly. The larger the placenta grows, the more food will be transferred to the baby. The weight of the placenta at birth is related to the weight of the baby, but the relation is not a close one. Some babies are born with placentas that are larger than would be expected from the size of their bodies. Why?

Shepherds have known for a long time that if they move pregnant ewes on to poor pasture in mid-pregnancy, and then return them to rich pasture in late pregnancy, the lambs are bigger than those of ewes who remain on rich pasture throughout pregnancy. This runs counter to common sense. Surely, a lamb will grow better if its mother remains well nourished throughout pregnancy. Recently Australian scientists have discovered how this works. When a lamb is undernourished during mid-pregnancy it increases the size of its placenta. It builds a bigger gate between itself and its mother. When the ewe returns to rich pasture, and food is more plentiful, the lamb uses this gate to get more food than it otherwise would have. But there is a catch. Although there is more food the baby has to share it with a larger placenta; and in the hierarchy of the womb the placenta dominates. Without the placenta the baby will perish. The lamb will grow better than it otherwise would but its size may not match that which would be expected from its large placenta.

Growth has costs. A larger placenta permits greater brain growth, but the price may be that more blood has to be diverted away from the rest of the body, whose growth suffers. If a mother is anemic, as millions are around the world, the baby receives less oxygen. Again the placenta responds by increasing its size, to extract more oxygen. Again there is a cost. The increased mass of the placenta requires more of the food available to the baby to sustain it.

Babies are like plants, which grow in different ways if they are well or badly nourished. Plants on good soil invest more of their resources in leaves and less in roots, so that they can use the increased energy obtained from more leaves to grow rapidly. Plants on poor soil invest in roots, in order to survive. Little is known about the way the human placenta responds to the mother's nutrition.

Little is known about the way the human placenta responds to the mother's nutrition.

While the baby thrives and grows, its placenta ages. The placenta dies at birth and is thrown away. What is discarded is not the remains of a worn out machine, built to genetic specifications to deliver itemised amounts of food to the baby. What dies at birth is a servant. To feed and protect the baby it has responded to the baby's commands. Hour by hour it has changed its transport systems, its barriers, the hormones it produces, to accommodate the changing world within the mother and nourish its master, the baby. It dies unmourned, and we know remarkably little about it.

NUTRITION IN THE WOMB AND LATER HEALTH

Much is known about the early growth of domestic animals. We know far more about the growth of pigs, sheep, cows and horses than we know about the growth of humans. Research into the growth of domestic animals fuels a large industry. Yet little is known about the long-term destiny of runt pigs or other animals that do not grow well in the womb. Their lives are brought to an end

We know far more about the growth of pigs, sheep, cows and horses than we know about the growth of humans.

Only now, with the emergence of research in which people are traced from birth to death, are we beginning to see the large impact of early growth and development on later disease.

long before they reach old age. Until recently, we knew little about the long-term destiny of small babies. They were born, cared for briefly in hospitals after which they dispersed into the general population. Only now, with the emergence of research in which people are traced from birth to death, are we beginning to see the large impact of early growth and development on later disease. Some social scientists find it difficult to accept that, when a child has been poorly nourished in early life, but is fed well later on, the biological legacy of its early experiences persists. It seems discouraging; but the reverse also holds. Biological advantages acquired by good experiences in early life persist despite later adversity. A good start is a foundation for a lifetime of health.

A good start is a foundation for a lifetime of health.

It is perhaps not surprising that inadequate feeding in early life is associated with chronic disease in later life, after reproduction is complete. The last chapter described how, when the food available to a living thing is limited, as it usually is, there have to be trade-offs. One part of the body has to be protected while another is sacrificed; one activity, growth, has to be achieved at the expense of another, repair. The less food there is the more trade-offs there have to be. We are beginning to understand the particular trade-offs that lead to later disease.

TRADING OFF THE KIDNEYS AND SETTING BLOOD PRESSURE

People in the town of Framingham, Massachusetts, have been studied for forty years or more. The study was among the first to show that people who develop heart disease have high blood pressure. The first suggestion that high blood pressure might have its origins before birth came from studies of Swedish military recruits, and from a continuing study of a group of British men and women who were all born during the same week in 1946. The pressure in a baby's circulation is critically important to it, because its nourishment depends on its ability to maintain an adequate pressure so that its blood flows freely through the placenta. A baby with a small placenta, that has narrow blood vessels, may need a higher blood pressure to maintain the   flow of blood through it. After birth these babies, who tend to be at the lower end of the birthweight range, continue to have higher blood pressures.

A baby with a small placenta, that has narrow blood vessels, may need a higher blood pressure to maintain the flow of blood through it.

At a fair, a palm reader looks at your hand and tells you your fortune. She examines the lines on your palms, the shape of your hands, and the patterns on your fingerprints. It is an entertainment: but we now know that it has a rational basis. The hands are formed early in pregnancy. The fingerprints are established around the nineteenth week of life. At birth undernourished babies tend to have 'whorls', complex patterns of ridges that are thought to result from their fingers being swollen when the skin is first laid down. People with whorls on several of their fingers tend to have high blood pressure. Undernourished babies also have narrow palms. People with narrow palms tend to have high blood pressure. Whether she knows it or not the palm reader is reading your life in the womb, and this determined your blood pressure today and may determine your health in the future.

Like children, babies respond variously to mal-nutrition, depending on its intensity, nature and at what age it occurs. Newborn babies who were thin or short and babies with small placentas have all been found to have high blood pressure in later life. Yet until middle age their blood pressures are only a little higher than those of other people,

Newborn babies who were thin or short and babies with small placentas have all been found to have high blood pressure in later life.

insufficiently raised to be a source of concern either to themselves or their doctors. It seems that even though a baby may be born with raised blood pressure it can maintain pressures within the normal range, preserve its internal constancy, the marker of good health, for many years. Eventually, as the system begins to wear out with age, this becomes impossible and blood pressure begins to rise steeply. When blood pressure rises, it damages the control systems, which include the kidney. The gentle rise in pressure that accompanies normal aging becomes a steep rise, a climbing pathway that leads to hypertension, increased risk of heart disease or stroke and the need for treatment. People who had low birthweight are twice as likely to need medicine to control their blood pressures towards the end of their lives.

People who had low birthweight are twice as likely to need medicine to control their blood pressures towards the end of their lives.

Within the human kidney there are at least a million functional units called nephrons, through which blood circulates so that the waste in it can be extracted. People who had low birthweights have up to three times fewer nephrons than people who were large at birth. The baby's kidney does not have high priority for growth because, in the womb, the excretion of waste is carried out by the mother's kidney. The baby's kidney is readily traded off. If, as a result, a kidney has fewer nephrons, once the baby is born each nephron will have to process more blood than it otherwise would have. This increases the wear and tear on them, and hastens the death of nephrons that occurs with normal aging. As nephrons die, blood pressure climbs, accelerating further nephron death and, it is thought, setting in motion a self-perpetuating cycle of rising blood pressure and nephron loss.

People who had low birthweights have up to three times fewer nephrons than people who were large at birth.

Nephrons are made during a brief period towards the end of life in the womb. If it were possible to make more nephrons after birth, kidney transplants would not be necessary. A review of the US Kidney Transplant program showed that the worst results, with failure of the transplanted kidney after only a few months, occurred when the kidney from a small person was transplanted into a large person. A large body has more blood to be cleared of waste, and the demand on each nephron is increased beyond its capacity. The nephrons die and the kidney fails. This may explain why people who had low birthweight are more likely to develop high blood pressure if they become overweight. Their nephrons die sooner and their journey to premature death is accelerated.

Kidney failure is commoner in South Carolina than in any other state in the US. It is usually preceded by high blood pressure or diabetes, but there are other causes. More men than women are affected, and people as young as 20 get it. To have kidney failure at so young an age is almost unheard off in many states. Many patients are poor, and the main burden falls on African-Americans in whom it is five times more common than it is among whites. We know all this because the costs of treatment, whether renal dialysis or kidney transplantation, are born by the Federal Government who keep accounts of what they spend and where they spend it. South Carolina is part of the so-called 'Stroke Belt', the cluster of states in the Deep South with high rates of stroke. Every baby born in the state since 1950 had its birthweight recorded on its birth certificate. It has therefore been relatively simple to show that people with kidney failure tend to have had lower birthweight. The high rates of kidney failure in South Carolina may be the result of an unusually large number of people being born with below average numbers of nephrons. If their kidneys are damaged by diabetes or other disorders they fail rapidly. The reasons why people in this state

> *Kidney failure is commoner in South Carolina than in any other state in the US.*

> *The high rates of kidney failure in South Carolina may be the result of an unusually large number of people being born with below average numbers of nephrons.*

have poor growth and development in the womb are the subject of Chapter 7.

TRADING OFF THE HEART

Until recently it was thought that the heart was not traded off. Like the brain it is essential for survival during development and is protected, though there must come a point beyond which protection is no longer possible. In the womb, as the heart pumps blood through the blood vessels in the placenta the pressures against which it has to work shape the thickness of its muscular walls and the size of its chambers for life. The mother's nutrition shapes the placenta; and the placenta shapes the baby's heart.

> *The mother's nutrition shapes the placenta; and the placenta shapes the baby's heart.*

At birth the heart is almost complete; its muscle cells are mostly mature and it needs only to enlarge as the body grows. Before birth it is sensitive to the environment. If it is undernourished it can speed up its maturation, perhaps in preparation for an early birth. This, however, leaves it with a smaller number of muscle cells, a diminished reserve for repair in later life. Another response, discovered only recently, is for the heart to slow its growth. But this too limits its reserve. People who had low birthweight have different hearts, for life. Many small babies are born with hearts that will be vulnerable to disease in later life. In order to maintain the supply of oxygen to the heart muscle the coronary arteries are swift to increase their size and number if they are challenged by low oxygen levels. In sheep even a few days of anemia, which reduces the supply of oxygen, remodels the coronaries in a way that, in humans, would protect against heart disease. This remodelling lasts for a lifetime. Though anemia in pregnancy puts mothers at risk is it ultimately beneficial to babies? Who knows? Whoever gave it a moment's thought?

> *Many small babies are born with hearts that will be vulnerable to disease in later life.*

TRADING OFF THE LIVER AND SETTING BLOOD CHOLESTEROL

Cholesterol is important because the body uses it to build the walls that enclose its cells. Most of the cholesterol in the body is not eaten in food but is made in the liver which controls how much cholesterol there is in the blood. A tape measure placed around the stomach of a newborn baby measures the size of its liver because, until it begins to feed, its intestines are mostly empty. There are large differences in the girth of the stomachs of newborn babies. This reflects differences in overall body size, but also the extent to which babies have traded off liver growth to protect brain growth. Remarkably, the girth of the stomach of newborn babies, reflecting the size of their livers, has been found to predict their blood cholesterol levels sixty and more years later. The greater the girth, the lower the cholesterol. We have become accustomed to the idea that high blood cholesterol, and the increased risk of heart disease linked to it, is evidence of an unhealthy diet. The truth may be that it is evidence of poor liver growth in the womb. In animals it is easy to change the activities of the liver permanently by altering the mother's diet in pregnancy. This happens because undernutrition changes the balance of the liver's specialist cells.

> *Most of the cholesterol in the body is not eaten in food but is made in the liver which controls how much cholesterol there is in the blood.*

> *Remarkably, the girth of the stomach of newborn babies, reflecting the size of their livers, has been found to predict their blood cholesterol levels sixty and more years later.*

After birth, the liver has to alter its function. Until that time it has been the first organ to receive and process the protein and sugars coming from the mother. After birth the baby's diet changes. It receives food only intermittently instead of constantly. Large amounts of cholesterol and saturated fat, the now forbidden foods of the western world, are taken into its body from the mother's milk and carried in the blood from the infant's intestines to the liver, where they are broken down and re-formed. Chapter 8 discusses whether these early experiences of cholesterol set the way the liver handles it for life.

TRADING OFF MUSCLE AND RESETTING BLOOD SUGAR

We think of insulin as the hormone which controls sugar, removing it from the blood and storing in the tissues, in muscle in particular, where it is used as a source of energy. But this simple housekeeping task is insulin's lesser role to which it is relegated after birth. Before birth it commands the baby's growth. It ensures that the speed of growth matches the availability of food.

People develop the common form of diabetes, which begins in adulthood, for two reasons: either their bodies do not make enough insulin, or their tissues, in particular their muscles, do not respond to it. Insulin is made by the pancreas in cells called beta cells. These beta cells develop before birth. In animals whose mothers were malnourished the beta cells do not function properly. They are less able to make insulin and meet the challenges of managing the body's sugar. One of these challenges is obesity, which makes the body less responsive to insulin, so that more of it is required. A reduced ability to make insulin, combined with an excess requirement for it, makes it impossible to maintain the amount of sugar in the blood at normal levels. The levels rise; diabetes develops.

Sensitivity to insulin is established in the womb. At any body weight people who were small at birth are more resistant to it than those who were large.

Obesity is not the only cause of loss of responsiveness, so-called "resistance", to insulin. Sensitivity to insulin is established in the womb. At any body weight people who were small at birth are more resistant to it than those who were large. It seems to be the thin, low birthweight baby that is most prone to becoming insulin resistant later. Like thin children, thin babies lack muscle though they may also lack fat. Run your fingers down the thigh of a thin newborn baby and you will readily feel the bone because the muscle is sparse. Muscle seems to have a low priority in the womb, and its growth is readily traded off if a baby is malnourished.

In the short-term resistance to insulin could be beneficial. If the muscles of an undernourished baby become resistant to insulin, more sugar will remain in the blood. This sugar will be available to the brain whose growth is thereby protected. Insulin resistance could be part of a system that enables the baby to be thrifty in its use of sugar. Priority is given to maintaining sufficient sugar in the blood rather than storing it in the muscles. Thrifty handling of sugar becomes 'hard-wired' and persists through life. It becomes a liability when food becomes more freely available after birth. The blood becomes flooded with sugar, and obesity makes the body still more resistant to insulin.

> *Insulin resistance could be part of a system that enables the baby to be thrifty in its use of sugar. Priority is given to maintaining sufficient sugar in the blood rather than storing it in the muscles.*

ADJUSTING TO STRESS

In the womb the hormone 'cortisol' controls the maturation of the lungs and of other systems that enable the baby to live independently of the mother after birth. It enters cells and turns on their specialized functions. There is a surge of cortisol as the time of birth approaches. When a baby is malnourished one option open to it is to increase its production of cortisol, mature rapidly and leave the womb prematurely. Like the tadpole in the drying pond, it can hasten its development and depart to a new life.

After birth, cortisol is part of the body's responses to stress, but these responses are less exalted than the maturation the hormone commanded before birth. They prepare the body for 'fight or flight'. Many animals use cortisol to adjust their internal environments to stresses in the external environment. In the breeding season the male Antechinus, a mouse-like animal, increases its cortisol production so that it can withstand the stress of repeated, intensive mating. The levels of cortisol become so high that, after the mating period, it dies, a victim of its own hormones!

People who were small at birth have more cortisol circulating in their blood and have a heightened response to stress for the rest of their lives.

People's levels of response to stress differ. People who were small at birth have more cortisol circulating in their blood and have a heightened response to stress for the rest of their lives. In the short term this may be unimportant, because the excess cortisol does not reach the levels that kill the male Antechinus. In the long term, it could be harmful. When cortisol is used as medication over many months, it raises blood pressure and produces insulin resistance. Smaller amounts produced by the body over many years, could have a similar effect.

It may not be the absolute level of life-threatening stress that is important in heart disease, but the response of the internal environment to what is perceived to be stressful.

For many years, a link between heart disease and stress was rejected. Heart disease is a recent disease that accompanies prosperity. Surely it could not be more stressful to be a factory worker in modern America, than a factory worker 100 years ago. We may have overlooked the fact that people respond to their perception of stress, or to symbols of stress. What is stressful to you may not be stressful to me. The swastika is a universal symbol. To Hindus and Buddhists it is a symbol of peace: to people who experienced the Nazis it is stressful. It may not be the absolute level of life-threatening stress that is important in heart disease, but the response of the internal environment to what is perceived to be stressful. Poorer people in America are not poor by world standards. They have food, homes and television sets. They are, however, at the lower end of a social hierarchy, and this may be stressful.

Men in the Helsinki study who have low incomes have more heart disease. It is however, only men who were small and thin at birth in whom low incomes have this effect. For men who were not thin at birth low incomes are without effect on heart disease. Perhaps only those people who grew slowly in the womb, and whose stress responses therefore became exaggerated, are susceptible to social stresses. This could be an important clue to understanding the worse health of poor people and ethnic minorities in the US.

Perhaps only those people who grew slowly in the womb, and whose stress responses therefore became exaggerated, are susceptible to social stresses.

This chapter leads to a general conclusion, though it is a tentative one that calls for more research. The internal environment of each individual is established in the womb and during infancy. Though it is based on a genetic blueprint, it is molded by the challenges of development. Among these challenges are matching the rate of growth to the availability of food, and when food is scarce protecting the growth of key organs by trading off the growth of other organs. Overcoming these challenges permanently changes the body, which is rendered more vulnerable to disease in later life. Reduced reserve capacity in organs such as the kidney and heart becomes critical as aging further reduces the reserve. An internal environment that uses food thriftily is harmful when food becomes abundant. Hormonal settings that are produced by the stress of malnutrition in the womb heighten the body's responses to stress in later life. Patients in hospitals and clinics may be paying

The internal environment of each individual is established in the womb and during infancy. Though it is based on a genetic blueprint, it is molded by the challenges of development.

the deferred costs of successful responses to the challenges of development—responses that enabled them to survive.

Summary

New research is showing why people who had low birthweight are more vulnerable to heart disease and diabetes. In the womb the heart has to pump blood through the placenta, and in small babies the high pressures in the placenta circulation weaken the heart for life. People who had low birthweight have fewer functional units in their kidneys and so tend to get high blood pressure. Their livers do not handle cholesterol efficiently. They are less responsive to insulin, and are therefore prone to diabetes. They are more readily stressed.

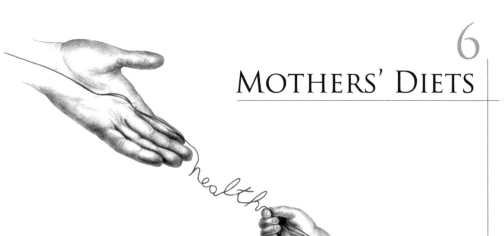

6
MOTHERS' DIETS

HOW A BABY GROWS IN THE WOMB is far more important than we had thought. So what should be done? A nutritionist Ronald McCance wrote long ago "the size attained in the womb depends on the services which the mother is able to supply. These are mainly food and accommodation." Of the two, food is more important to the baby's lifelong health.

How a baby grows in the womb is far more important than we had thought.

WHY DO PREGNANT WOMEN NEED TO EAT?

When, during the Second World War, Allied paratroopers failed to establish a bridgehead at Arnhem in western Holland, Hitler ordered the occupying forces to take revenge against the Dutch people, who had aided the allies. Tight restrictions on food supplies were imposed and official rations fell to starvation levels. Old people died, babies were stillborn, many women ceased to menstruate. But the birthweights of babies who were already in the womb when the famine began fell, on average, by only ¾ pound. Which raises the question why do pregnant women need to eat at all? Some mammals—bears, seals—do not eat during pregnancy.

One answer is that although the babies in wartime Holland were able to grow, they were lastingly changed by their experience in the womb. For a baby growth is a high priority. If it does not grow a sufficiently large body it will perish when it is born. But in a malnourished mother it grows at a cost. It has insufficient resource to establish strong organs and systems, or an internal environment that will be resilient to stress when it enters the world beyond the womb. Another reason for eating during pregnancy is that mothers expend energy and will become thin if they do not eat, which is what happened to the mothers in Holland. As the next chapter describes, this of itself will create problems for the baby, who needs the protein and fat that are stored in the mother's muscle and fat and released into her blood each day.

THE WOMB IS NOT A PADDED CELL

Because babies seem able to grow to reasonable size, almost independently of what the mothers eats in late pregnancy, the view has developed that the baby in the womb is a highly successful parasite, like a tick or a leech, able to take from the mother whatever it requires, and satisfy its modest needs. For as long as the baby is in the womb, the argument runs, it is able to fend for itself, and it is only after birth that it becomes vulnerable. In the womb the baby is protected, buffered from the world by the mother's body, a shield pierced only by poisons or dangerous infections. Alone in its cell it lives out its genetic potential to be greeted at birth with cries of "It's got father's chin, mother's eyes." Such a comfortable picture is far from the true one. The baby is sensitive to what is happening outside its warm pool. Every pulse of its mother's blood brings to it a various and varying supply of foods. These shape its structures and its systems.

The baby is sensitive to what is happening outside its warm pool. Every pulse of its mother's blood brings to it a various and varying supply of foods. These shape its structures and its systems.

DIET BEFORE PREGNANCY

A baby does not live only on what the mother eats during pregnancy. It also depends on the food stored in her body. Animal breeders have always known that ewes, mares, sows and cows need to be well nourished before mating so that their offspring grow well in the womb. In human breeding it has become the custom for mothers to become concerned about their diets only when they know that they are pregnant. This curious view may have arisen because, in the past, giving food to malnourished pregnant women and children in industrial cities was a focus of charitable activity. Because the embryo and fetus are small in early pregnancy it was assumed that undernutrition at the time of conception was not a problem, and the needs of malnourished adolescent girls were neglected

> *A baby does not live only on what the mother eats during pregnancy. It also depends on the food stored in her body.*

We now know that the fetus responds to the mother's diet and food stores from the beginning of pregnancy. Assisted reproduction, developed to help infertile couples, has shown that we humans are the same as the animals among whom we live. Assisted reproduction is widely practised in farm animals. When eggs are removed from a female and fertilized outside her body the composition of the fluid in which the eggs are kept can alter the rate at which the baby grows. Human babies fertilised in test tubes tend to be small.

> *We now know that the fetus responds to the mother's diet and food stores from the beginning of pregnancy.*

Lack of food slows growth long before the fetus runs out of building blocks. If, from the time of mating, sows are given food that is low in protein, the piglets are already small in mid-pregnancy. Some are smaller than others as competition for food between brother and sisters begins early. Undernutrition must therefore slow growth through processes other than the simple lack of building blocks with which to make the body. These processes are controlled by the baby's hormones. Insulin is the most important of these. When a mother reduces her food intake, the baby reduces the amount of insulin it makes, which slows its growth. Insulin and hormones like it give the baby the ability to match the rate at which it grows to the availability of food. When food is scarce the baby is able to slow its growth in a coordinated way, and does not have to wait until the building blocks are exhausted and further growth becomes impossible. Such an event would have serious long-term consequences for whatever parts of the body were growing rapidly at the time.

> *When food is scarce the baby is able to slow its growth in a coordinated way, and does not have to wait until the building blocks are exhausted and further growth becomes impossible.*

In animals the embryo responds to its mother's nutrition even before it implants in the wall of her womb, which in humans occurs on the eighth day after fertilization. When the protein in the diet of female rats was reduced for a brief two-day period around the time of mating, the structure of the embryos was visibly changed at a stage of development when they were no more than hollow balls of cells. At birth they were small but after birth they grew rapidly and developed raised blood pressure for life. Another astonishing consequence of early nutrition is the birth of giant farm animals. When test tube techniques were first introduced into animal breeding, lambs of twice the normal size began to appear. Giant calves were born with giant hearts. Such profound, life-long changes in response to transient early experiences show how sensitive the embryo is to its mother's nutrition. Perhaps this is not surprising. While a living thing consists of only a few cells, the entire body which it will become can be altered. Later on only those parts of the body that are at 'sensitive periods' of development can be changed.

There is no reason why the egg should only begin to respond to the mother's nutrition when it is fertilized. While the egg matures in the first two weeks of the menstrual cycle it could be changed by the nutrients that reach it. This line of thought leads on to ideas which, until recently, were seldom articulated. Since a girl is born with all the eggs she will ever release will the quality of the eggs be reduced if she is undernourished while still a child? Was the quality of your body, and therefore your health through life, established by the food that your mother's mother made available to your mother when your mother was laying down the egg that made you?

This leads to two conclusions. First, women need to be on a good diet before they become pregnant. Second, the growth and nutrition of girls may be more important to the health of the next generation than we have suspected. This is discussed in the next chapter.

> *First, women need to be on a good diet before they become pregnant. Second, the growth and nutrition of girls may be more important to the health of the next generation than we have suspected.*

WHY NOT TRUST OUR INSTINCTS?

The composition of a good diet was agreed in America almost a hundred years ago and it remains agreed today. The diets of many Americans, however, are unbalanced and monotonous. The US Department of Agriculture (USDA) reports that people eat too much fat, too little fruit and too much sugar and salt. They eat too limited a variety of vegetables so that half of all vegetable servings are iceberg lettuce, potatoes or canned tomatoes.

If a woman recognizes that her diet is less nutritious than it might be, why cannot she simply rely on instinct to improve it? The answer appears to be that while people around the world eat many different foods, human beings do not innately know how to choose a nutritious diet, and tend to prefer diets that are sweet and fatty, and foods that are dense in energy.

WHY NOT RETURN TO A TRADITIONAL DIET?

There is no traditional American diet. Take a walk through your local supermarket. You will probably enter through the fruit and vegetable section. There will be potatoes, a staple food but a recent one, until a few centuries ago growing only in the high Andes. There will be maze which is traditional and sustained the Native American civilizations; but it is a nutritionally deficient food which, eaten alone, leads to Vitamin B$_3$ deficiency. There will be pears, apples, plums and peaches—all foreign foods introduced by the settlers from Europe. On nearby shelves there will be bread made from wheat, another foreign food introduced to make the barren lands of the Great Plains habitable. And there will be cornflakes, invented a hundred years ago by a fanatic who believed that fiber and roughage would suppress lust. At the fish counter the oysters are truly an ancient American food, the nearest thing we have to 'natural' food, eaten alive, uncooked; but the salmon are farmed. At the meat counter at least the sausages are in a traditional form, the best of them still stuffed into tubes made from innards. But the beef is from animals that were introduced into America simply because they were easy to herd and there is no wild meat, no hares or turkeys or buffalo or venison. Butter will be difficult to find, but there will be many margarines, even though margarine originated in response to the need for grease to maintain firearms, and only became a food when Napoleon III offered a prize for "a product suitable to replace butter for the less prosperous classes of society." There will be shelves of processed foods, designed only to be tasty and predictable. There will be foods like hamburgers, which were introduced by the food giants to provide cheap, hygienic food. Some of them will be fortified with vitamins, whose origins lie in science but which became a craze. "Vitamins will win the war," was a Second World War slogan.

> There is no traditional American diet.

CAN SCIENCE HELP?

Around the world people eat many different foods and there are many different diets which promote good health and long life. In 1917 USDA issued a pamphlet entitled "How to select foods". It divided foods into five groups, fruit and vegetables; meat and other protein-rich foods; cereals and other starchy foods; sweets; and fats. It described in simple terms how these five food groups met the body's needs for growth, maintenance and work. It did not recommend any particular foods or combinations of foods. Over the years nutritional science has brought a more detailed understanding of how the body handles food, but has not changed the USDA recommendations.

The recommendations were used to form the widely known pyramid of five food groups. At the base are the foods obtained from plants - bread, cereal, rice, pasta, fruit and vegetables. Above are foods obtained from animals—meat poultry, fish, eggs, dairy products—recommended to be eaten in lesser amounts than the foods below. At the apex are fatty and sugary foods, to be eaten sparingly. The strength of this picture is that it is simple, widely agreed, describes basic foods, and represents a more healthy diet than most people actually consume. It remains the basis for a good diet today, but now has a scientific basis.

For people looking to improve their diets some understanding of this science may be helpful. But detailed knowledge of the nutrients contained in each food, and the daily requirements for each nutrient, the currency of modern dietetics, is unnecessary and confusing. A varied diet provides the necessary nutrients, and people's daily needs vary widely. A diet that meets all the needs can be created without weights and measures. Scientific principles do not exclude beliefs about food that arise from religion or culture and the USDA recommendations accommodate a wide range of tastes and preferences. The essentials of the five food groups are readily summarised.

Breads, cereals, rice and pasta are the carbohydrate foods that form the foundation on which a diet is built. How much of them are needed is largely determined by a person's energy requirements, a product of his or her body size and level of physical activity. There is a mistaken belief that these foods make people fat, and some weight-reducing diets recommend their avoidance. The fact is that they are no more fattening than any other food eaten in excess.

Meat is not an essential component of the human diet even though it has formed a significant part of it for thousands of years. Meat, fish, poultry, eggs, beans and lentils all provide protein. Whereas carbohydrates are the body's energy source, proteins form the structure of the body, making up about one sixth of its weight. Much of this is muscle, but there is also protein in the body's organs and in the skin. Proteins are also part of the body's transport system: like boats they carry nutrients, hormones and other messengers through the channels and canals of the body. They are made up

The amount of protein foods required depends on how much carbohydrate food is eaten.

from amino acids, of which there are around twenty different kinds. Each amino acid has different functions and capabilities. Like the letters of the alphabet, they can be joined together in many different ways to give a rich vocabulary. 'Non-essential' amino acids are those that can be manufactured in the body. 'Essential' ones must be supplied by foods. Meat, fish, poultry and eggs each contain all of the necessary essential amino acids, and the profile of amino acids in each of them is similar and close to what nutritional science regards as desirable. Beans and lentils are good sources of protein; but different types tend to be low in particular amino acids, which argues for eating a variety. The amount of protein foods required depends on how much carbohydrate food is eaten. The recommended balance of the amount of protein to carbohydrate is around one portion of protein food to two portions of carbohydrate.

Five servings of fruit and vegetables a day have become widely accepted as desirable and attainable. There is no prescription for the kind of fruit or vegetables or the balance of one to the other. They carry little risk of obesity, because they are low in energy. They contain many vitamins, as well as minerals drawn from the soil. They are also a rich source of anti-oxidants, the body's protection against oxygen. Even though it is essential for life, oxygen causes damage. Rust is the result of damage to metal by oxygen. In the body cell walls are damaged by their constant exposure to oxygen.

Fruit and vegetables contain so-called 'soluble' fiber, which is digested. Cereals, including breakfast cereals, contain 'insoluble' fiber, which is not absorbed but increases the speed with which food passes through the gut. There is a belief that this rapid passage of food is beneficial, but the evidence which supports this is fragmentary. The prominence of insoluble fiber in discussions of diet may owe more to the profits made from it by the food industry than to its biological importance.

Green leafy vegetables have been shown to increase babies' birthweights. They have a greater effect on birthweight than would be expected from the growth-promoting substances, such as folic acid and iron, that they are known to contain. This suggests that they contain beneficial substances, minerals or vitamins, that have yet to be identified. The existence of such substances could explain why, when mothers

Green leafy vegetables have been shown to increase babies' birthweights. They have a greater effect on birthweight than would be expected from the growth-promoting substances, such as folic acid and iron, that they are known to contain.

take supplements of single nutrients, such as zinc, the benefits for their babies are disappointingly small. It argues for eating a variety of fruit and vegetables, an argument that is reinforced by the wide variation in the amount of vitamins and minerals contained in different types of fruit and vegetables.

Milk is a rich food. Milk, and milk products such as cheese and yogurt, provide around three-quarters of the calcium in an average American diet, and have been an important part of traditional diets since animal farming began. During pregnancy the mother has to transfer around one ounce of calcium to the baby. She achieves this by making more calcium available to the baby from the substantial reserves in her bones. Although health messages about the possible links between dietary fat and heart disease have led to recommendations that skimmed milk is preferable to whole milk, there must be uncertainty as to whether this advice is wise for young women. Skimming removes more than fat: vitamins are dissolved in the fat and removed with it.

While carbohydrates are the baby's immediate source of energy, and proteins form the substance of its body, fat is used to make the walls that separate one cell from the next one. Towards the end of pregnancy the baby begins to accumulate fat. This serves as an energy store for the period after birth when milk feeding has to become established. After birth the baby builds up a second store of fat, in preparation for weaning, when the food supply becomes uncertain. Fats are built up from fatty acids. Whereas there are only around twenty different amino acids, the range of fatty acids is much greater. Like amino acids, some fatty acids can be manufactured by the body, but others are 'essential' and must be supplied by food, particularly oily fish, meat and eggs.

Towards the end of pregnancy the baby begins to accumulate fat. This serves as an energy store for the period after birth when milk feeding has to become established.

The pattern of fatty acids in our cell walls determines our ability to respond to the environment. This is one of several scientific reasons for eating a variety of fatty foods. Fatty acids contain hydrogen, and the more hydrogen they have the more 'saturated' they are. Different fatty acids, with different levels of saturation, have different properties. Saturated fats have been linked to the development of heart disease and, though the evidence is inconclusive, the general advice is to avoid large amounts of foods with high saturated fat content. Fatty acids, however, are important structural components of the baby's brain, so health messages about the suspected long-term dangers of fat consumption should not create a barrier to the baby receiving adequate fatty acids. Fats in the food also bring with them vitamins A, D and E, which dissolve in fat but not water, and are therefore not present in large amounts in foods such as fruit and vegetables.

> *Fatty acids, however, are important structural components of the baby's brain, so health messages about the suspected long-term dangers of fat consumption should not create a barrier to the baby receiving adequate fatty acids.*

A SPECIAL DIET FOR PREGNANCY?

There are no scientific reasons why a woman who is eating a good diet when she conceives needs to alter her diet during pregnancy, other than avoiding a few foods such as liver, which contains too much Vitamin A, and soft cheeses, which can carry infections. In this way her diet during pregnancy will become the diet onto which her child is weaned. The way a baby is nourished in the womb establishes how it handles food after birth. If it is poorly nourished it handles food frugally, and may be less able to adjust to higher food consumption later on. As described in the last chapter the muscles of malnourished babies become resistant to the effects of insulin, which conserves the sugar in their blood

> *The way a baby is nourished in the womb establishes how it handles food after birth.*

NUTRITION IN THE WOMB

but makes them unable to maintain normal blood sugar levels if they become even modestly overweight in adult life. It is possible that if food is over-abundant in the womb, because the mother changes her diet and consumes more of some foods, the baby may develop a wasteful metabolism, so that it comes to depend on high levels of nutrients being available. After birth it might become deficient in vitamins or minerals at levels of food consumption that would be adequate for people with a more economic metabolism. Only experiments on animals support this disquieting notion; but it raises doubts about the wisdom of taking large amounts of supplements during pregnancy. It supports the general thesis that women need not change a habitual good diet when they become pregnant.

...women need not change a habitual good diet when they become pregnant.

THE BODY'S FOOD FACTORY

The human body is not just a furnace, capable only of consuming food and needing regular stoking with anything that will burn. It is a re-fashioning and a re-cycling plant. You can make yourself a tasty supper of meat, potatoes, herbs and vegetables, and then share it with your dog. You will change the food into more of you, while your dog will make it into more dog. Your supper, however, will probably fit your needs better than the dog's. There is a television game show in which two teams are given access to a pile of scrap metal from broken down machinery, and are asked to construct a new machine, a crane, a hoist, a cart. It is a test of ingenuity, but crucial to success is whether the scrap metal contains materials that fit the requirements of the machine the teams are trying to make. In the same way, it is easier for your dog to use your supper if the food happens to fit its particular needs.

The human body is not just a furnace, capable only of consuming food and needing regular stoking with anything that will burn. It is a re-fashioning and a re-cycling plant.

The teams that are building the machines do not depend solely on the good fortune of finding scrap that matches what they need. They can modify the scrap metal to make it fit their needs. Our bodies can do this. We have systems that enable us to refashion the food we eat and live healthily off different diets. An example of these systems is our ability to manufacture amino acids. A baby needs a large amount of different amino acids, as building blocks and as a source of energy. Some amino acids cannot be manufactured in the body and are therefore essential components of the diet; but others can be made, by refashioning what is in the diet. Women enter pregnancy with a greater or lesser capacity to refashion food for the benefit of their babies. Taller, larger women generally have more capacity than small women. Differences in mother's refashioning capacity explain twenty-five percent of the differences in birthweight between babies. At present it is not possible to measure refashioning capacity, though there is no fundamental reason why, at some point in the future, family physicians will not have simple tests for this.

Differences in mother's re-fashioning capacity explain twenty-five percent of the differences in birthweight between babies.

THE BODY'S RECYCLING PLANT

The teams in the television game are recycling waste. Humans have their own internal waste re-cycling plant, in the colon. Its activities depend on bacteria. Nature depends on bacteria to rot down and dispose of waste. Bacteria have a seemingly infinite ability to break down all kinds of matter. Those in the colon not only break down food, they also reform it into useful substances—vitamins, fatty acids, amino acids. They live on the fiber from fruit and vegetables (but not breakfast cereals), on other undigested food, on the secretions of the gut and on the dead cells sloughed off from the wall of the gut. They make the colon a fermentation chamber that is important in meeting the body's need for food.

In the past the body's needs were calculated simply from what the food of seemingly healthy people contained. We now know that this seriously underestimates what is required. The body's needs are now calculated by measuring its demands. For example, as part of the daily consumption of protein, an adult eats around 800 milligrams of the amino acid lysine. The body, however, demands more than twice as much. If we attempted to make up this shortfall by doubling our consumption of protein, the increased need for meat and soybeans would have catastrophic global economic and environmental consequences. Happily, the colonic bacteria solve this dilemma. They use the nitrogen from waste products to make up the shortfall.

More Protein is not Necessarily Better

Forty years ago an obstetrician set up a practice in a steel town in Scotland. Many of the families in the town were on low wages, and foods rich in protein were expensive. At that time preeclampsia, a common illness in pregnancy that threatens the life of both mother and baby, was thought to be the result of lack of protein. To prevent this disorder the obstetrician encouraged the town's pregnant women to eat a pound of red meat every day. In a booklet given to each expectant mother, he wrote, "quantity of meat is more important than quality. As it may be difficult to eat enough meat at mealtimes the use of cooked meat, especially corned beef, rather than fruit or biscuits, is advised to assuage hunger between meals." He discouraged mothers from eating foods that were rich in carbohydrate, because excessive weight gain in pregnancy was also thought to be linked to preeclampsia. "Do not eat potatoes or chips, or bread—either white, brown, malted or toasted—or rolls, scones, cakes or biscuits of any kind."

The birthweights of babies born in the town fell. A similar fall in birthweight had been found in other places where pregnant women were given extra protein, including in New York when poorer women were given protein supplements. When some of the Scottish babies, now grown up, were recently examined their blood pressures were raised. The more meat their mothers had eaten, the higher their blood pressures. If their mothers had eaten few green vegetables, the blood pressures were even higher. What had gone wrong?

It was a manifestation of a general phenomenon that extends beyond birth. In the months after birth a baby gains weight at a faster rate than it will at any later age, and much of the weight gained will be protein. Yet breast milk contains less protein than will be consumed in the diet at any later age, and extra protein as a supplement will make the baby unwell. Against what seems to be common sense, the best diet to make a baby grow is not a diet packed with protein.

> *Against what seems to be common sense, the best diet to make a baby grow is not a diet packed with protein.*

Enzymes control the processes by which the amino acids in proteins are refashioned and recycled. In order to function these enzymes need folic acid and B vitamins, whose natural sources include bread and potatoes. The Scottish mothers were specifically advised to avoid these two foods. They therefore had a reduced capacity to make new amino acids. The large amounts of meat in their diets provided an excess of essential amino acids. These are potentially toxic unless they are broken down. Breaking them down uses up non-essential amino acids, which are required for the process. The availability of non-essential amino acids to the Scottish babies was therefore reduced both by the mother's reduced capacity to make them, and by their diversion to breaking down essential amino acids. The baby's' growth had to slow.

In another Scottish town, at around the same time, the diets of a group of pregnant women were recorded in an attempt to discover what particular foods were linked to their babies' birthweights. Some of the women were poor and, by today's standards, had small amounts of protein in their diets. Their babies tended to have low birthweights, especially if the mothers ate a lot of carbohydrate foods. Their low protein diets provided too few building blocks for their babies to grow, while the high carbohydrate diets provided the energy for growth but not the materials. There were plenty of bricklayers, but too few bricks..

The experiences of pregnant women in these two Scottish towns show that there is a desirable balance in the amount of protein eaten in relation to the amount of carbohydrates. Too much protein or too little have harmful effects. High protein, low carbohydrate diets are popular aids to slimming because breaking down the protein uses up energy.

Too much protein or too little have harmful effects.

BALANCE

At one level the need for a balanced diet seems obvious, but when people say "it's better to have a little of everything rather than a lot of one thing" they are talking about variety, not balance. Balance is about harmony; and there is more than one kind of dietary harmony. Traditional societies had to establish a harmony between what food their immediate surroundings could provide and the way their bodies used particular nutrients. In parts of West Africa people have very low intakes of calcium, but their bodies retain and use it economically. The body also has to harmonize the energy it spends maintaining itself and moving around with the provision of energy from outside. What one part of the body needs another part must provide and the two activities must harmonize. The amino acids needed to maintain the protein in muscle depend on the activities of the colon, which in turn are fuelled by the soluble fiber in fruit and vegetables.

The high meat diet in the Scottish town upset the balance between the manufacture of amino acids and their disposal. The average American needs 4 grams of salt a day, but takes in 10, mostly in refined foods. The excess is disposed of in urine; but potassium is inevitably disposed of with the sodium, and the stores of potassium within the body, which come from fruit and vegetables, are depleted. So the large amounts of salt in processed foods waste the benefits of fruit and vegetables.

VARIETY

People on the island of Crete consume three times more fat than Americans but, at the time of the Seven Countries Study, Americans had forty times as much heart disease as Cretans. Much of the fat eaten in Crete is raw olive oil, which has led to years of research into why vegetable fats appear to be less harmful than animal fats. Nevertheless, the low rates of heart disease in Crete remain largely unaccounted for. If there was evidence that olive oil reduces the risk of heart disease to the almost non-existent risk there once was in Crete, the manufacturers of olive oil would proclaim it and everyone would consume the oil in large amounts.

The USDA recommendations did not single out particular foods as good and others as bad. The riddle of Crete will not be solved by identifying a single life-saving food, but by characterising Cretans overall diet. To do this it is necessary to know something of their history. Until the middle of the seventeenth century Crete had close ties with the Greek mainland. But from 1669 until 1898 the island was ruled by the Turks. The ties with the Greek mainland were

The USDA recommendations did not single out particular foods as good and others as bad.

severed and Cretans were reduced to living off foods that could be obtained locally, through cultivation, hunting and the exploitation of wild plants. After the Turks left, Cretans continued to get their supplies from local sources, and their cuisine remained seasonal. Even today there are few wild plants that are not used in cooking.

Cretans eat three times as much bread as the average American and twice as much fruit. They grow apricots, peaches, pears, grapes, oranges, not in large farms but in gardens, and the taste and texture of the same fruit, and therefore their mineral and vitamin content, varies across the island. Cretans eat a variety of beans, lentils and vegetables, including wild vegetables such as chicory, artichoke, wild tomato and cucumber, purslane, notch weed and black nightshade. A Cretan eats greens, beans and lentils every day, but never eats the same food on one day and the next. Dairy products are important in their diet.

The Cretan diet is characterized by variety. Today even a simple lunch in an inexpensive taverna is likely to include many different foods. At one such I recorded a meal of artichokes, cucumber, beetroot, red pepper, celery, wild greens, olives, potatoes, egg, lamb, pork, shrimp, yoghurt, apples, oranges, kiwi fruit, nuts and bread. This was neither a large nor a heavy meal. The next day, at the same place, there were similarly small portions of aubergines, courgettes, onions, tomatoes, cabbage, lettuce, potatoes, pork, two kinds of small fish, cherries, lemons and bread. Such a varied diet is an insurance against deficiencies in nutrients, both those that are known and those that science has not yet identified. We can live off a varied diet because our refashioning systems permit this. We can convert one food into another but we cannot make up for deficiencies in essential nutrients. In the Third World people eat unvaried diets, and suffer from deficiencies of minerals and vitamins, because they have no other choice. In the US people choose to eat unvaried meals.

Historically, with the introduction of farming the diets of societies that had depended on hunting and gathering became less varied. Some societies came to rely on a single staple food, on rice, wheat, rye or potatoes. Restriction of the diet brought with it more dangers of famine and disease. Dependence on a single variety of potato drove a million Irish people to America when a fungus wiped out the crop. Early settlers in the US had neither abundance nor variety. At times the settlers in Virginia depended for their survival on food given to them by native people. Survival on the Great Plains was only possible because cattle could survive on wretched land, and technology turned wasteland into wheat fields. Cretans have had a varied diet for centuries. For Americans it is a new possibility.

> *Cretans have had a varied diet for centuries. For Americans it is a new possibility.*

FOOD CHOICES

I recently met a young woman who says she lives on pasta and coffee. Her diet sustains her from one day to the next in her busy life, but it will not meet the demands that any illness will bring; she is unlikely to succeed in sports; and she will not be able to meet the challenges of pregnancy. So why does she eat in this way? Perhaps she is trying to lose weight. Perhaps the pace of her life is such that there is no time to cook. Perhaps she does not come from a culture where eating is a social activity, and she bolts down her dismal meals in the isolation of her apartment. Or perhaps she does not know the customs of choosing, preparing and cooking food that are familiar to older people.

When people are asked why they do not eat a better diet they often reply that there is not enough time in the day to prepare and cook

...for many young women the phrases 'healthy eating' and 'dieting to make me slim' are inter-changeable.

food. This may be a perception rather than a reality. People usually make time to do things they regard as important. Another commonly given reason is that for many people a good diet is less palatable than a bad one. Most people do not perceive lack of knowledge about food as a barrier to eating a healthy diet. In a recent survey, 70% of people across Europe believed they were eating a healthy diet! One source of confusion is that for many young women the phrases 'healthy eating' and 'dieting to make me slim' are interchangeable.

Consumers may need to understand how they are being manipu-lated, if the epidemics of heart disease and diabetes are to be brought to an end.

Shopping for a healthy diet should be a simple matter. Semi-literate peasants in southern Europe have done it successfully for centuries. The food industry, however, has made food shopping complicated. The industry has successfully made hygienic food available to everyone in abundance, but to make profits it has had to manipulate food choices. Across America there are 320,000 different food items competing for supermarket shelf space that can hold only 50,000. Consumers may need to understand how they are being manipulated, if the epidemics of heart disease and diabetes are to be brought to an end. The manipulations include price, supplementation, fortification and labelling.

PRICE

In order to maintain their profits food companies need to add value to basic foods. They process, freeze, can and pre-package them. The corn in a packet of cornflakes costs less than ten percent of the price! Processed foods are useful because they enable busy people to prepare appetizing meals quickly, but over-reliance on them brings the risk of deficiencies or excesses of particular nutrients. Seventy percent of new foods are convenience foods.

Despite this food prices in the US are low by world standards. The average American pays less than ten percent of his or her income on food. Yet price increases are strongly resisted, and lower prices stimulate sales. One in four British people say that price is an important barrier to eating a better diet. Only one in ten French or Italian people share this view. The British reply is curious because the monotonous, unbalanced diets they often eat are expensive. They are also poor value for money. Sugary foods, for example, contribute little nutritionally. For an Italian, eating is culturally important, a social occasion rather than simply refuelling. Meals are not just pit stops but something worth spending money on. The quality of food matters to them.

To many Americans the quality of food seems unimportant. In the canteen of the National Institute of Health in Washington the food one selects is priced simply by how much it weighs! One of the leading American airlines now economizes on food costs by giving each passenger what they call a 'Bistro Bag' when boarding the plane. Bistro is a European word for a place where people meet to talk, laugh, enjoy the company of their friends, drink wine and dine on home-cooked food. To equate a processed turkey roll in a paper bag with a Bistro may be a stretch too far!

FOOD SUPPLEMENTS AND FORTIFICATION

One half of all the people in the US take supplements of vitamins, minerals or herbs. The belief that these are a kind of nutritional insurance is irrational, given the wide availability of basic foods; but these products are strongly promoted by their manufacturers. Under current law the manufacturers can make claims for health benefits for which scientific support may be limited, dubious or non-existent.

> *One half of all the people in the US take supplements of vitamins, minerals or herbs. The belief that these are a kind of nutritional insurance is irrational, given the wide availability of basic foods...*

73

All they are required to do is to avoid claims that are inherently misleading, and to not sell supplements that are harmful. Not only is the use of supplements irrational but it is beginning to emerge that supplements have unexpected hazards because they by-pass the body's normal handling processes. Iron supplements intended to prevent anemia may end up feeding pathogenic bacteria in the intestines! Supplements to food, and fortification of food with vitamins and minerals, have a role to play in improving nutrition in the Third World. It is hoped that this will be a temporary role, an expedient while improved agriculture and better food distribution become established.

In the US both supplements and food fortification thrive because the public is encouraged to focus on the health benefits of single nutrients. The media assist in this. Further scientific evidence that fruit is good for the heart will not be widely reported, but "new studies show that vitamin E prevents heart attacks" (or impotence, or ageing, or hair loss) will be reported everywhere. In the past food fortification was helpful. Adding iodine to salt prevented goitre. Today fortification is mostly unnecessary. Fortification with iron seems to be one of the exceptions. Yet one quarter of all new food products are nutritionally enriched. Pause between mouthfuls of corn flakes and wonder why corn, a staple food of humankind for centuries, now in this time of abundance has to be enriched.

In the twentieth century nutritional science identified, one by one, disorders which resulted from deficiencies of single nutrients, beginning with vitamins and continuing with essential amino acids, essential fatty acids and most recently trace elements. Treatment of these disorders had spectacular effects, producing swift and permanent cures of a kind only equalled in today's medicine by antibiotics and hormones. Entire communities were restored to health. Within the lifetime of many Americans pellagra, a disabling disease caused by lack of Vitamin B$_3$, which affected tens of thousands of people in the southern states, has disappeared.

These discoveries set fashions. The science of dietetics grew up, emphasizing the different nutrients contained in each food. Books for pregnant women listing each component of every food multiplied. They gave, however, a false sense of prescription; they implied, wrongly, that measurement and accuracy are required. The amount of a particular nutrient that is needed depends on the foods being eaten and on refashioning activity, which varies from one person to another. Recently folic acid has become a focus for women planning to become pregnant. Lack of it leads to spina bifida. Women are being advised to have extra folic acid before conceiving. In so far as this will prevent a rare congenital disorder this is prudent, but folic acid has many functions in addition to its specific ones on closure of the spinal column. It is, for example, essential for refashioning processes. The use of folic acid supplements, and the fortification of food with folic acid, remain debatable issues. People argue that since "folic" comes from the word "foliage", or leaves, why do we not deal with the problem by eating more leaves.

> *The amount of a particular nutrient that is needed depends on the foods being eaten and on refashioning activity, which varies from one person to another.*

LABELLING

Why is any food labelled? Fresh food is not labelled. The labels on processed foods, showing what they contain, may seem to offer a safeguard to consumers, but this is an illusion. A former Commissioner of the Food and Drugs Administration wrote that labels had become "so opaque or confusing that only consumers with the hermeneutic abilities of a Talmudic scholar can peel back the encoded layers of meaning. This is because labels spring not from disinterested scientific reasoning, but from lobbying, negotiation and compromise." Labels undermine the good intentions of consumers. Labels such as 'healthy', 'natural', 'balanced' are meaningless.

WHAT YOUNG WOMEN EAT

Keeping a diary of the food eaten over a number of days is one obvious way to find out whether what you eat corresponds with what you think you eat. A diary kept for one day represents a snapshot of a diet that may change from day to day, but research shows that even one-day snapshots broadly reflect peoples' habitual patterns of eating. When young women have been asked to keep food diaries, the problems with their diets have been obvious. Some eat vegetables and salads but no fruit or dairy products. Dieting to lose weight brings difficulties. If chicken is the only source of protein, and dairy products are largely avoided in the belief that they are fattening, there may be an inadequate variety of fats. Vegetarians sometimes rely too much on processed foods, such as vegetarian sausages and nuggets, rather than beans and lentils as meat alternatives.

First, many young women in the US eat unbalanced and monotonous diets, but their daily meals could easily be modified to resolve this. Second, increasing the variety of foods would take care of imbalances and deficiencies in minerals and vitamins.

Studies of the diets of young women regularly lead to two conclusions. First, many young women in the US eat unbalanced and monotonous diets, but their daily meals could easily be modified to resolve this. Second, increasing the variety of foods would take care of imbalances and deficiencies in minerals and vitamins. The only common exception to this is iron, which women lose through menstruation. The rich sources of iron are meat and green vegetables, which some women do not eat, but bread and breakfast cereals are fortified with iron.

Summary

A baby does not live only on what the mother eats during pregnancy. It also depends on the food stored in her body. Within days of conception the human embryo is sensitive to the nutrients it receives from its mother. Therefore women need to be on a good diet before they become pregnant. The composition of a good diet was agreed in America almost a hundred years ago but the diets of many Americans today are unbalanced and monotonous. The balance of protein to carbohydrate is important: too much or too little protein is harmful to the baby.

The rate of heart disease in the US is forty times higher than it is in the Greek island of Crete, where the diet is characterized by variety. Cretans have had a varied diet for centuries. For Americans it is a new possibility, but people still choose to eat unvaried meals.

The human body is not just a furnace, capable only of consuming food and needing regular stoking with anything that will burn. It is also a re-fashioning and recycling plant. Women enter pregnancy with a greater or lesser capacity to refashion food for the benefit of their babies. Shorter women have a lesser capacity.

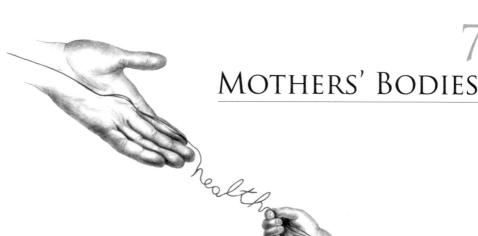

7

MOTHERS' BODIES

BABIES BORN TO THE SAME MOTHER, but by different fathers, tend to have similar birthweights. Babies with the same father, but different mothers, have different birthweights. Studies of domestic animals show that it is the mother who controls the size of the baby. In a famous experiment small Shetland ponies were crossed with large Shire horses. The foals were smaller at birth when the Shetland pony was the mother than when the Shire horse was the mother. As the genetic composition of the two crosses was similar the body of the Shetland mother must have constrained the growth of her foal.

> *Studies of domestic animals show that it is the mother who controls the size of the baby.*

Large women tend to have large babies. They have a greater capacity to refashion food and they provide more spacious accommodation in the womb. A new technique to help infertile couples is for an egg to be donated by another woman, fertilized in a test-tube by the husband's sperm and then placed in the wife's womb. The birthweight of the baby will be related to the wife's body size, but will not be related to the size of the woman who donated the egg. The mother's body size is more important than the baby's genes.

THE FOOD STORES IN A MOTHER'S BODY

If a baby in the womb depended only on what its mother ate each day it would be too vulnerable to the mother becoming temporarily short of food or ill. Many pregnant women lose their appetites or have long periods of sickness. Rather than being dependent on her daily diet the baby calls on the mother's food reserves. These reserves are nutrients that have accumulated before pregnancy and are stored in particular parts of the body, for example iron in the bone marrow, folic acid in the liver. Another reserve is the protein, fat and calcium that are incorporated into the mother's tissues, her muscle, fat, and bone.

If a baby in the womb depended only on what its mother ate each day it would be too vulnerable to the mother becoming temporarily short of food or ill.

The body is like a beehive. Its fixed external shape conceals a dynamic state of breakdown and renewal within it. Muscle, fat and bone are broken down each day, releasing protein, fat and calcium which are then re-incorporated back into the tissues. This is called 'turnover'. It is an important source of food for a baby as the mother is constantly enriching the nutrients in her blood from the stores in her own body. This allows her to adapt to different foods and varied activities. It's the same flexible system that is now used for money. In olden days banks kept money locked up in safe deposits: today they constantly turn it over, investing, selling, and reinvesting.

Each day a young woman breaks down and renews three percent of her muscle. The amount of amino acids circulating in her bloodstream, and therefore available to her baby, will be influenced by the rate and scale of her turnover. Mothers with more muscle and larger organs can more readily make amino acids

Each day a young woman breaks down and renews three percent of her muscle.

available to the baby. Thin mothers have lower rates of turnover. The mother's turnover and her diet work in harmony. The relative importance of either of them depends on circumstances. In the war-time famine in Holland the mothers' bodies were almost the only source of protein.

The body's fat stores are also turned over each day. In women, fat makes up about one third of the body's weight. Although it is most apparent where it is stored under the skin, there are hidden stores in the cavities of the abdomen. While only about one percent of a mother's fat stores are turned over every day, the size of the stores is such that the fatty acid composition of a mother's diet during pregnancy may only be of secondary importance. Bone turns over continuously, forming and reabsorbing, taking in calcium and releasing it into the blood. Turnover increases in pregnancy, so that the baby's bones are constructed from the calcium in the mother's bones.

> ...the baby's bones are constructed from the calcium in the mother's bones.

BABIES DEPEND ON THEIR MOTHER'S LIFETIME NUTRITION

Women who have low birthweight babies tend to have had low birthweight themselves. Long ago Edward Mellanby, famous as one of the discoverers of Vitamin D, wrote that "it is certain that the significance of correct nutrition in child bearing does not begin in pregnancy itself or even in the adult female before pregnancy. It looms large as soon as a female child is born and indeed in its intrauterine life." An anthropologist, Ashley Montague, wrote, "A mother's good nutrition over her whole lifetime results in the superior development of her own body. If she has grown normally from her own prenatal days her own organs will be splendidly equal to the job of nurturing her child; if not they may be less able. On the other hand, a young woman whose own background has been poverty-stricken or deprived can, by providing a good diet for herself and her child, compensate to a large extent for her deficiencies." This was written many years ago, and the author can have had only a general idea of what might be the "deficiencies" that a young woman from a deprived background brings to pregnancy. Among the candidates are a lesser ability to refashion food, a restriction on the size of placenta that the baby is able to build and short stature which, like the small Shetland mare, will constrain the baby's growth.

THE SIZE AND SHAPE OF MOTHERS

A woman's lifetime nutrition is reflected in her body size and shape. Around the world the size and shape of girls and young women varies widely and is changing rapidly. This must have profound consequences for the growth of babies. The average weight of young women of a comparable age is 90 pounds (41 kg) in rural India and 141 pounds (64 kg) in the US. Even within Western countries girls and women have a remarkable range of body weights. In Britain the weights of 16-year old girls living in the same city were found to range from 77 to 213 pounds (35 to 97kg).

Fatness is assessed by the weight of the body in relation to the height, the so-called body mass index, weight/height^2. The body mass index of the 16-year old British girls ranged from 15 to 35. A body mass below 18 is regarded as thin, but is average among young women in rural India, where many girls are poorly nourished from childhood. In Western countries many girls and young women are as slim as this by choice. Current advice is that women with a body mass index below 18 could usefully gain weight before becoming pregnant, providing they do so on a balanced and varied diet. A person is defined as overweight if their body mass index is above 25, and obese if it exceeds 30.

Current advice is that women with a body mass index below 18 could usefully gain weight before becoming pregnant, providing they do so on a balanced and varied diet.

Although a high body mass index may also be a result of muscularity it more often results from fatness. The problems associated with obesity in young women are well known, and the period before pregnancy may be an appropriate one in which to try and reduce fatness.

The problems associated with obesity in young women are well known, and the period before pregnancy may be an appropriate one in which to try and reduce fatness.

Women store fat in different places, and fat stored in different parts of the body has different actions. Fat on the arms, below the shoulder or above the hips makes different amounts of estrogen. Overweight women whose fat has accumulated on the abdomen are resistant to the effects of insulin, a problem not shared by those who store fat on their hips.

In the US, women gain around 26 pounds (12 kilograms) in weight during pregnancy. 17 pounds (7.7 kilograms) of this is due to increase in fat, in fluid and in the tissues of the womb and breast. Pregnant women accumulate around 7 pounds (3 kilograms) of extra fat in the first half of pregnancy. This provides an energy store for the second half of pregnancy when the baby's need for energy is greatest, and when it is building up its own fat stores in preparation for birth. Although there are recommendations for desirable levels of weight gain in pregnancy it is difficult to control. A woman who eats a balanced diet may be best guided by her appetite.

Thin women tend to have small babies, who are resistant to insulin and therefore predisposed to diabetes in later life. The levels of thinness at which this happens are not extreme but those encouraged by the fashion industry. This is not widely known. A recent article in a New York magazine describes how thinness and

Thin women tend to have small babies, who are resistant to insulin and therefore predisposed to diabetes in later life. The levels of thinness at which this happens are not extreme but those encouraged by the fashion industry.

avoidance of weight gain in pregnancy has become an obsession. "Going home from the hospital in the same jeans you wore before you got pregnant becomes a symbol that you're still the same person you used to be!"

Fifty years ago in China, while Mao Tse-tung was camped with his army in the Fragrant Hills, waiting to enter Beijing, work at a hospital in the city continued undisturbed. The Peking Union Medical College Hospital was brought by the Rockerfeller Foundation in 1920. The Foundation's vision was to create a school where the brightest of China's medical students could be trained. Doctors were brought from the US to teach them, and a modern hospital was established. As part of their obstetric training the students attended the delivery room and were required to make detailed observations on each newborn baby. These included taking the baby's footprints and making drawings of the placenta, in ink, showing both its surface and its appearance from the side! These were added to the copious notes which were begun when the mothers first came to the hospital in early pregnancy, and which included their heights and weights.

Around the time China's Civil War finally came to an end, in 1949, 600 babies were born in the hospital. They were born and were lost, disappearing into the new Communist world of a billion people, living through famine and the Cultural Revolution, before settling again in Beijing where, a few years ago, they were traced by Chinese researchers wishing to examine them. As expected the people who had been thin or stunted at birth were resistant to insulin and more of them had diabetes. But those born to thin mothers were at especially high risk. Their mothers' low turnover of protein and fat may have made them less able to nourish their babies adequately. Other studies in the US and Europe have since confirmed this link between maternal thinness and diabetes in the next generation.

MALNOURISHED MOTHERS IN US HISTORY

Today it is overweight not thin women who are the focus of concern about the well-being of future generations. Both thinness and overweight are the result of malnutrition. The children of overweight women are also at increased risk of diabetes, though through different processes than those which affect the children of thin women. Rather than being resistant to insulin they have difficulty making it. The children of overweight mothers who were themselves malnourished as children, and are therefore short in stature, are at greatest risk of later disease. The geography of diabetes, heart disease and stroke across the US today was laid down by the undernourished mothers of the past. Overweight mothers will fuel the epidemic of chronic disease in the next generation.

> *The children of overweight women are also at increased risk of diabetes, though through different processes than those which affect the children of thin women.*

> *The geography of diabetes, heart disease and stroke across the US today was laid down by the undernourished mothers of the past. Overweight mothers will fuel the epidemic of chronic disease in the next generation.*

Many of the immigrants in the USA in the 1800's and early 1900's came because they were destitute. Two hundred years ago the average calorie intake in Europe was similar to that in poorer parts of Africa and India today. At such low levels of food consumption many starved, and people's capacity for physical work was low. The great improvements in European health over the next two centuries were founded on improvements in agriculture and a steep increase in the supply of food, what the Chicago economist and Nobel Laureate, Robert Fogel, has called 'the escape from hunger'. While this was happening one way for an individual to escape from hunger was to go to America. Among the masses who reached the US some were fleeing persecution, but most were escaping hunger and destitution. Though they no longer starved many, in factory towns and poor farms, continued to be poorly nourished. The story of the cotton mills of New England is an illustration.

In 1810, Francis Lowell travelled from New England to Lancashire, England to examine and memorize the textile machinery that had been invented for the thriving Lancashire cotton industry. Lowell remarked on the large numbers of women employed in the mills. Spinning and weaving were peculiarly suited to women, or rather girls, because they demanded neat hands and dexterity. On his return to New England, he built cotton mills and others soon followed his example. The girls who came to work the looms in the new textile cities of Lowell, Lawrence, Manchester, Nashua, and in towns along the Saco River Valley in Maine, came from nearby family farms. They came to escape a narrow and confined life, and to earn money. Though in the mill towns they slept two to a bed, they were well fed and encouraged to continue their education after working hours.

Over the years, as the owners sought to increases their profits, wages fell and conditions deteriorated. In his book, 'The Belles of New England', William Moran quotes a worker's letter to a mill owner, published in a local paper around 1840. The letter said the girls were being robbed of their health just at the time they were coming into full physical maturity. "Your factory system is worse by far than that of Europe: you shut up your operatives two or three hours longer a day in your factory prisons than is done in Europe." The letter wrote of frequent uterine prolapse, miscarriages and stillbirths.

The women began to leave the mills. The owners hired men to recruit more. The men travelled to the depressed rural areas of Maine, New Hampshire, Vermont, and loaded onto their wagons women who were desperate to escape. "There are hundreds of young females shipped from this State every year to the factory prison-houses", wrote a Maine newspaper, "like cattle, sheep and pigs sent to slaughter". As wages fell further, immigrants came to the mills, from Ireland, Poland, Italy and Greece. The mills advertised in

European villages, "No-one goes hungry in Lawrence. Here all can work, all can eat." In 1912, when the workers in Lawrence went on strike, a New York newspaper described it as an industrial blot on the map, a place where human beings were starved in order to produce vast wealth for the mill owners "a city of hunger and destitution, of child labor, of women labor." Some of the cotton mills in the South were no better. Undernourished little girls of seven worked from 6 in the morning to 7 at night.

A hundred years ago half of all the 11 million wives in the US lived on farms, and all but the youngest had spent their youth in heavy manual work, taming the wilderness. One million women worked in factories: a disproportionate number of them were young, an immigrant or the daughter of immigrants. Today millions of Americans have maternal grandmothers who were undernourished and overworked in their youth and mothers who, as a consequence, were small at birth and tended to remain short. This prejudiced the early growth and lifetime health of the next generation, today's Americans. Those whose mothers had low birthweight and were short are at the highest risk of chronic disease. In this lie hitherto unsuspected explanations for the distribution of diabetes, heart disease and stroke in the US today. Because America is a mobile society studies that link geographical differences in the rates of chronic disease to past geographical differences in the nutrition of young women are difficult to do. It is easier to establish the existence of these links in Europe.

> *Today millions of Americans have maternal grand- mothers who were undernourished and overworked in their youth and mothers who, as a conse- quence, were small at birth and tended to remain short.*

MOTHERS' LIFETIME NUTRITION AND HEART DISEASE

During his visit to Lancashire Lowell commented on the poor physical condition of many of the women who worked in the mills. His visit is likely to have included three important cotton-weaving towns. Burnley is in a valley: Nelson and Colne lie on the hillside above it. Today there is hardly a break in the lines of houses between one town and the next. Many people are employed as manual workers: and living conditions and lifestyles in the towns are similar. Yet there are large differences in the rates of heart disease in the three towns. In Burnley the rates are 20 percent above the national average, making it one of the least healthy towns in the country. Rates in Nelson, however, are around the average, while in Colne they are intermediate between the other two towns. History offers an explanation of this.

One hundred years ago almost half of all the women and girls in the three towns worked in the mills. In Burnley and Colne many of the women were from the second or third generation of Lancashire industrial workers, and had grown up in tiny houses in crowded streets. The houses were damp, especially those in Burnley which were built in a marshy valley and were made even damper by water leaking down from the canal embankment above them. Some houses were built 'back-to-back' with no means of ventilation to the outside air. In these conditions many infants suffered from recurrent bronchitis and pneumonia. The houses were also unsanitary, and lacked facilities for the storage of food and milk. Infantile diarrhea was common. In 1912 one in every four babies born into these back-to-back houses died before reaching the age of one year.

The young women who grew up in these conditions, and went to work in the mills at the age of 10, were stunted. When their babies were born they too were small and many died. Many mothers had to return to full-time work just a few days after having had a baby. Usually the mother's return to work was followed by complete weaning and the infant, together with other children in the family below school age, was placed in the care of an untrained "minder" paid for by the mother.

Nelson developed more recently than Burnley and Colne. Most of its people were immigrants from nearby rural areas. "This fact," wrote a report in 1914, "has an important bearing on the question of infantile mortality, owing to the general good health and the habits of cleanliness and thrift characteristic of these immigrants from rural districts." The women were described as "sturdier and healthier" than those in Burnley and Colne. Among the children and grandchildren of the stunted mothers in Burnley, heart disease is common. Among the children of the country girls in Nelson the disease occurs at no more than average rates. Heart disease is Burnley's legacy from a century of malnourished girls and young women.

The early origins of heart disease are intimately linked to the growth of the placenta. Some people who develop the disease had small placentas; others had large placentas in relation to the size of their bodies, suggesting that the transfer of food across the placenta was inefficient and it had to enlarge to compensate. The growth of the placenta depends upon the nutritional state of the mother. Perhaps succeeding generations in Burnley receive their blighted inheritance through poor placental growth.

In the U.S. as in Britain heart disease is a legacy from malnutrition and poor living conditions among previous generations of girls and young women. It is a legacy generated by the industrial revolution and by settlement on barren lands that gave meagre returns to the families who farmed them. Has any western country escaped this legacy?

> ...heart disease is a legacy from malnutrition and poor living conditions among previous generations of girls and young women.

Sit in a restaurant in southern France, watch the cigarette smoke rising above the nearby tables, read the list of rich foods on the menu, marvel at the variety of alcoholic drinks, and wonder why France has much lower rates of heart disease than the US. A Nobel Prize winner once wrote that, "For every complex problem there is a simple, easy to understand, incorrect answer." Until now, only simple and easy to understand explanations, such as red wine and garlic protect against heart disease, have been brought forward to explain the "French paradox". Not surprisingly, these simple ideas have not stood the test of time.

In 1871, the German army reached the gates of Paris. This demoralizing defeat in the Franco-Prussian War made the French fear that their army was physically inadequate and that France would cease to be a military power. These fears were compounded by concerns about the diminishing numbers of children in the country, as a result of the low birth rate and high infant mortality. Over the next thirty years various measures were introduced to protect the nutrition and health of the country's children. After the turn of the century the medical journal, the Lancet, sent a representative to Paris to report on France's programs for mothers, infants and children. He found that a meal (soup, meat and vegetables) was being provided free to every schoolchild. In both Paris and the provinces there were infant welfare centers promoting breast-feeding and, when this failed, providing sterilized cows' milk from milk depots. Local communities, 'communes', established after the Revolution provided an organizational framework within which national directives could be translated into local action. Communes took responsibility for the welfare of pregnant women.

A feature of industrialization in the US was that the wages that enticed men and women into the factories were often received at the cost of their children's nutrition and well-being. The dense inhabitation of towns and cities, with the frequent infective illnesses that accompanied overcrowding in the home, stunted children's growth. In some places, such as coal mining towns, where family survival depended on the manual labor of men, boys were given more

> *A feature of industrialization in the US was that the wages that enticed men and women into the factories were often received at the cost of their children's nutrition and well-being.*

and better food than girls. The nutrition of young women in factory towns and poor farms may have been further impaired by early marriage and large families. The French may have largely escaped the epidemic of heart disease by focussing improved nutrition on mothers, babies and young children, and by making each community take responsibility for the welfare of pregnant women and infants.

> *The French may have largely escaped the epidemic of heart disease by focussing improved nutrition on mothers, babies and young children…*

MOTHERS' LIFETIME NUTRITION AND STROKE

The word 'stroke' is used to describe damage to the brain resulting from lack of blood when arteries burst or become blocked. Like heart disease it is a result of hardening of the arteries and high blood pressure. For more than half a century strokes have been more common in the southeast of the USA than anywhere else in the country. The so-called 'stroke belt' comprises a contiguous cluster of states in the southeast, with South

> *For more than half a century strokes have been more common in the southeast of the USA than anywhere else in the country.*

Carolina as the focus. High death rates from stroke affect men and women, blacks and whites, with especially high rates in young blacks. High blood pressure is also more common in the 'stroke belt'. Despite intensive investigations over many years there is no agreed explanation for the existence of the belt. There seems to be no common lifestyle differences that would explain it, and neither do differences in medical care offer an explanation.

There are, however, two clues. The first comes from South Carolina which for decades has had the highest death rates from stroke in the United States, with rates 50% to 60% above the national average. Within the state stroke is most common among people who were born there; it is less common among those born elsewhere in the southeast; and least common in those born outside the southeast. To be part of the stroke belt you have to be born there. This conclusion is supported by findings among black people in New York. As a group they have high death rates from stroke, but these high rates are confined to people who were born in the southern states.

The second clue to the stroke belt is that within the belt the highest death rates are in people with poor education, low incomes and unskilled occupations. Among affluent people there is no excess of stroke mortality in the southeast, no stroke belt. The two clues suggest that stroke originates before birth, and is therefore linked to mothers, and specifically to mothers from poor backgrounds. There is important new evidence on this. The Helsinki studies, introduced in Chapter 3, show that the mothers of men and women who had high blood pressure and suffered a stroke had small pelvic bones, indicated by a reduction in several standard diameters of the pelvis, which can be measured externally using callipers. One of these diameters, the so-called external conjugate, measures the front to back size of the pelvis, specifically the distance between the pubic bone, situated behind the pubic hair, and the back of the lowest vertebrum in the spinal column. Other pelvic diameters measure the width of the pelvic bones, from side to side, at different levels. In the past the pelvic bones were routinely measured at antenatal clinics to assess the likelihood of obstructed labour.

Small pelvic bones are a persisting consequence of undernutrition during infancy, in particular lack of Vitamin D. This softens the bones and slows their growth. Its greatest effect is on the external conjugate. When an undernourished infant with soft bones begins to stand, the forces on the bony pelvis tend to flatten it from front to back. The external conjugate diameter is reduced, and this persists as a lifelong marker of undernutrition during infancy. While the pelvic bones continue their growth during childhood and adolescence the proportions of the pelvis, front to back versus side to side, are not remodelled. A woman who was undernourished during infancy reaches the ante-natal clinic with a clear record of this, a "flat" pelvis. Being born to a mother with a flat pelvis was one of the strongest predictors of stroke in the Helsinki study. The side to side measurements of the mother's pelvis did not predict stroke. This points to a specific effect of undernutrition and poor growth during the mothers' infancy.

Therefore to understand the US stroke belt we need to go back to the childhoods of the mothers of people now getting strokes. This is a one century backwards leap to a time when malnutrition was widespread among people living in the stroke belt. The social disruption which began in the Civil War and continued until the depression brought with it food shortages and vitamin

> *Therefore to understand the US stroke belt we need to go back to the childhoods of the mothers of people now getting strokes.*

deficiencies. The deficiency disease pellagra, in which people have chronic diarrhea and skin troubles and become demented, remained common among poor people in the south until the 1930s. Their diets of pork fat and 'hominy grits' made from corn were deficient in vitamin B3. In those times of hunger and vitamin deficiency infants in poor families would have been especially vulnerable.

Reared in poverty, with short stature and flat pelvices, mothers in the stroke belt were at risk of dying during childbirth, from difficulties in giving birth, from haemorrhage, from toxaemia. In western countries death rates among mothers during childbirth remained at a disturbingly high level well into the twentieth century. It was described as "a deep, dark and continuous stream of mortality." Women with poor physique were more likely to die in childbirth than taller, sturdier women. In Britain today the strongest predictor of the rates of stroke in any one place remains the death rates among mothers around seventy years ago.

In Britain today the strongest predictor of the rates of stroke in any one place remains the death rates among mothers around seventy years ago.

Mothers in the southern states had babies who were vulnerable to stroke in their later lives. They may have been vulnerable because the blood vessels in their brains were poorly developed, and weakened with advancing age so that they burst or became blocked. One explanation of why mothers reared in poverty are less able to nourish their babies is that they have an impaired ability to refashion food. A woman's ability to re-fashion the food she eats is built up through her life, but her dietary experience before birth and during infancy seem to have the greatest impact on it. Women, who were poorly nourished at this time may have a more limited repertoire of refashioning activities and a diminished response to the extra needs of pregnancy. During pregnancy a key aspect of refashioning is the ability to re-constitute the proteins obtained from food into those that better fit the baby's needs. The continuing high rates of low birthweight in the stroke belt may reflect the persistence down the generations of a refashioning ability that became compromised by events more than a century ago.

One explanation of why mothers reared in poverty are less able to nourish their babies is that they have an impaired ability to refashion food.

The continuing high rates of low birthweight in the stroke belt may reflect the persistence down the generations of a refashioning ability that became compromised by events more than a century ago.

Beyond the severe degrees of pelvic flattening which rendered women liable to obstructed labor and death, there were lesser deformities. The advent of X-rays around 1930 allowed obstetricians to study the shape of the female bony pelvis in close detail.

The major focus of numerous reports was a search for the optimal shape of the so-called pelvic inlet, the bones surrounding the upper end of the birth canal, the first obstacle which the baby's head encounters. Was childbirth easier if the inlet was oval from side to side or was it easier if the inlet was round. A study at Yale compared the inlets of a group of nurses with those of patients in an antenatal clinic. The nurses, who came from comfortable backgrounds, had rounder inlets than their patients, who had grown up in poorer homes. This and other evidence led to the round pelvic inlet being declared as superior. Every woman has, in the size and shape of her pelvic bones, a permanent record of her nutrition during infancy and childhood.

> *Every woman has, in the size and shape of her pelvic bones, a permanent record of her nutrition during infancy and childhood.*

SUMMARY

A baby's growth does not depend only on what its mother eats each day. That would make it too vulnerable to the mother becoming temporarily short of food or ill. It is nourished by it's mother's muscles, fat and bones. Protein, fat and calcium are released from them each day and then re-incorporated back into the tissues. This process, 'turnover', constantly enriches the mother's blood. A woman's turnover, and her ability to refashion food, are built up in response to her dietary experiences through her life. Experience in early life seems to have the greatest impact and short women have a lesser capacity to refashion food.

Thin women tend to have babies who are resistant to the action of insulin and are therefore predisposed to diabetes in later life. The children of overweight mothers also have an increased risk of diabetes. The geography of diabetes, heart disease and stroke across the US today was laid down by the undernourished mothers of the past. Short, overweight mothers will fuel the epidemic of chronic disease in the next generation.

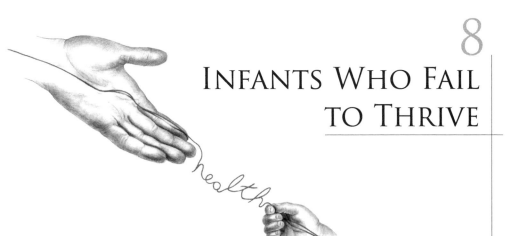

INFANTS WHO FAIL TO THRIVE

8

AFTER IT IS BORN A BABY RESPONDS differently to malnutrition. No longer receiving food and oxygen through blood returning from the placenta, it has to readjust its circulation so that it can receive food through its intestines and oxygen through its lungs. Much of the body is complete. Organs like the kidney are beyond their sensitive periods of development and are no longer vulnerable.

The next phase of growth is infancy, which lasts from birth to two years of age. Though both the length and weight of a baby increase rapidly in the first months after birth, it also grows fatter. Most babies double their birthweight in the first five months. This is usual: no one knows if it is optimal. Thereafter, growth slows: by one year the birthweight has tripled. At the age of six months fat makes up a quarter of the body's weight. After this age there is a gradual decline in fatness and proportionately more muscle is deposited. The fat laid down in the first six months provides an important store of energy for the infant to use during weaning, as at this time eating behavior is unreliable. By the age of around

> By the age of around 2 years, when childhood begins, the height an infant has attained predicts its final adult height...

2 years, when childhood begins, the height an infant has attained predicts its final adult height, just as the size of the shinbone of a foal predicts the final size of the horse.

The new interest in infant growth that has been generated by its links with later chronic disease has revealed major gaps in our knowledge. One of them is our ignorance about what governs growth from the time of weaning to two years of age. As in the womb, growth during infancy ultimately depends on the supply of food, but it is also sensitive to its surroundings. Poor living conditions will slow it's growth. Infections such as diarrhoea and bronchitis spread readily in unsanitary, overcrowded households, and to combat them an infant has to divert energy away from growth. People grow more rapidly during infancy than they do at any later age. Almost one quarter of the energy available to an infant is used for growth, which makes growth vulnerable to the body's other demands for energy.

Almost one quarter of the energy available to an infant is used for growth...

While many people are able to find out what their birthweight was few are able to discover how they grew as infants. The long-term consequences of infant growth are therefore known in less detail those of growth in the womb. Nevertheless the general picture, from Hertfordshire, Helsinki and elsewhere, is clear. Slow weight gain during infancy, leading to a child who is stunted or thin at the age of two, increases the risk of high blood pressure, heart disease, stroke and diabetes in later life.

Slow weight gain during infancy, leading to a child who is stunted or thin at the age of two, increases the risk of high blood pressure, heart disease, stroke and diabetes in later life.

For much of the body, birth brings an end to plasticity, but two large organs, the brain and the liver, together with the immune system, remain plastic for some years after birth. The brain and the lymphoid tissue, part of the immune system, are the tissues that grow most rapidly during infancy. At birth, the brain cells are in place, but many have not yet been connected. The connections are not closely specified by genes. The network that comes into being as the brain grows is too complex to be under genetic instruction. Rather it is evoked by the stimuli the baby receives from its surroundings. Michael was not necessarily born to be intelligent, manly or withdrawn; he became so largely through experience. "Give me a child until he is 7 years old and I will give you the man" wrote the Jesuits.

Infants who grow slowly tend to achieve less at school and during their working lives. This could be the result of poor brain growth, but undernourished babies also reduce their movements in order to conserve energy. In the slums of South America listless, sickly babies lack the energy even to disperse the flies that swarm upon them. By restricting their movement they receive less stimulation from their surroundings, which holds back the development of their intelligence.

> *Infants who grow slowly tend to achieve less at school and during their working lives.*

After birth bacteria colonise the baby's intestines. This process begins moments before birth when the baby, who has never encountered bacteria, enters its mother's vagina. There, for the first time, it meets the bacteria which will form the flora of its intestines for the rest of its life. The gut of a newborn baby is like an incubation chamber and bacteria settle in rapidly. They will fuel the colonic recycling plant, described in Chapter 6, which synthesises new foods from what would otherwise be the body's waste. Intestinal colonisation begins in the vagina, continues whenever the baby is fed and is completed after weaning. Thereafter there are more bacteria in the gut than cells in the body. Within the gut there is a living jungle;

> *Within the gut there is a living jungle; a stable ecosystem that lasts for a life-time.*

a stable ecosystem that lasts for a life-time. Our unique personal gut flora is one of our lasting inheritances from our mothers. We may have underestimated how important this inheritance is for it seems to have powers that are as yet unknown. Animals that are kept free of bacteria do not become obese if they are overfed. The kind of bacteria acquired from the mother at birth differs around the world. Bacterial DNA is now being used to study the origins of peoples.

One skill which an infant is not able to learn from its mother is how to respond to the bacteria and viruses it encounters. The mother's accumulated experience of this does not inform the baby, who has to learn how to respond for itself. The dilemma is that while it needs to acquire experience, in order build up its barriers, it must avoid being overwhelmed. Large size at birth and breast feeding assist in this. The thymus, the lymphoid tissue in the neck which controls immunity, is larger in large babies and in babies who are breast-fed. There are also bacteria in breast milk which may play a role in educating the baby's immune system, but little is known about this.

> *One skill which an infant is not able to learn from its mother is how to respond to the bacteria and viruses it encounters.*

In the Gambia, in West Africa, there is a time of the year known as the "hungry season". This is the time at the end of the dry season. Food has become scarce; the rains bring mosquitoes and malaria; and women have to labor in the fields, digging up the land before planting new crops. Babies' birthweights fall and children die. Those who survive are prone to getting infectious diseases throughout their lives. As adults they have higher death rates than people born in other seasons. Research has shown that babies born in the hungry season have small thymuses. The thymus develops just before birth and an undernourished baby will trade off thymic growth in order to conserve energy and survive. There is, however, a long-term cost. The immune system is weakened and the body becomes vulnerable to infections.

In ways that are little understood the growth of an infant is influenced not only by the food it receives but also by its experiences before birth, which set its hormones and metabolism and determine how it responds to food. There is not one path of growth that is optimal for every baby. It depends on the baby. Because knowledge of this is limited mothers may receive contradictory advice. A number of different aspects of development accompany growth, gain in height, increase in muscle and fat, development of cognitive function and of physical and psycho-social skills. It is possible that there are trade offs. Rapid weight gain may be good for the development of the brain but in some circumstances could increase the risk of obesity in childhood. More research should resolve these uncertainties. Happily the larger picture is encouraging. Infants who grow well are healthier, more intelligent and more productive in later life. No one is advocating the promotion of infant growth by over-feeding. Rather the goal is the protection of infants by good feeding and by freedom from recurrent infectious illness.

In ways that are little understood the growth of an infant is influenced not only by the food it receives but also by its experiences before birth...

There is not one path of growth that is optimal for every baby. It depends on the baby.

BREASTFEEDING

Mammals are distinguished by the way they nourish their young after birth. The female frog rapidly completes her investment in her offspring and abandons the tadpoles within a mass of nutrient jelly. A bird invests in the egg and then does no more than sit on it. After hatching, it has another chance to nourish its young, but the system is a clumsy one. The parents must leave the young for long periods, days even, exposing them to predators and other dangers. The newborn mammal, however, simply reattaches itself to its mother: the breast replaces the placenta.

Through pregnancy, in the networks of signalling between baby, mother and placenta, there are many different dialogues. In later pregnancy one dialogue is between the placenta and the breasts. Hormonal signals from the placenta prepare the breasts for lactation. In experiments in rats where part of the placenta was removed less breast milk was available to the young after birth, so that they grew more slowly than they otherwise would. Perhaps the placenta gives the breasts advance notice of the size of the baby and therefore its likely needs for milk. The breast responds by ripening an appropriate number of milk ducts. Excess milk production is wasteful, using energy which the mother needs for herself.

Newborn mammals can find and attach themselves to their mothers' breasts without her assistance. Bears, whether brown, black or polar, mate in the spring. The embryo's growth is then suspended through the summer until autumn, when it implants in the womb and begins to develop. Almost immediately the mother ceases to feed and enters a den, where she spends the winter hibernating, without food or water. While she sleeps her cubs are born and begin breast-feeding. She awakes to greet her suckling infants.

There is no debate that breastfeeding provides ideal nourishment for the human baby, and that the act of suckling helps to bond a mother and baby psychologically. Breast milk provides sufficient energy, nutrients and fluid for at least the first four months. It also contains a repertoire of hormones, growth factors and antibodies. The hormones and growth factors promote the growth of the baby's intestines. The antibodies protect the baby from infections. In the evolution of mammals, and in the early life of a woman, the breast began as skin, whose function is to protect the body from infection. The mother's breast retains this function, preventing inflammation in the baby's gut and thereby protecting its growth. Though the stomach of a newborn baby is no bigger than its mother's fingertip, and can take only small amounts of milk, even a few weeks of breastfeeding confer lasting benefits.

If it is so widely agreed that breastfeeding is the best way to nourish a newborn baby, why is it that in some western countries only a minority of babies are fed this way? In the US 68% of babies are breastfed at birth; 31% at 6 months. Rates vary markedly from one place to another, even between different parts of the same city. Culture and custom sometimes discourage breastfeeding. In coal-mining areas, for example, the sexual needs of men employed in dangerous and demanding jobs used to take precedence over the needs of the baby. Breastfeeding was perceived as conflicting with the sexual role of the breasts. This perception is part of other, older cultures. Mende women in Sierra Leone soon take their infants off the breast and give them tinned milk instead. They, and other peoples in West Africa, believe that a man's semen contaminates breast milk and may make the infant sick. Sexual intercourse cannot be resumed until breastfeeding ceases, and early resumption is important to the mother because it helps bond her with the father, on whom she is economically dependent. Today, in many countries, the need for improved workplace facilities for breastfeeding mothers remains an issue. Sweden has demonstrated that changes in attitudes to breastfeeding in the workplace and across society can lead to huge increases in breastfeeding—from 20 percent among two-month old babies in 1973 to 85% twenty years later. Although all mammals successfully accomplish breastfeeding, some women become discouraged by early problems. Many young women in the US know little about breastfeeding. In the past a girl would see her mothers, aunts or cousins feeding their babies. Today, some young women are repelled even by the notion of it.

Bottle Feeding

Some mothers wish to breastfeed but are unable to do so. Happily, although the healthy baby fed exclusively on breast milk for the first four to six months remains 'the gold standard', a mother who chooses to bottle-feed can purchase "infant formulas" with considerable confidence. Cows' milk is unsuitable for young infants because it places too great a burden on the kidneys. Modern formulas, in which the content of the milk has been modified, provide satisfactory substitutes for human milk. The law now requires that infant formulas satisfy the nutritional needs of babies while not providing an excess of any nutrient. The protein in them must come from cow's milk or soy protein. Given that many elderly people alive today were fed on condensed milk, or on other unsuitable substitutes for breast-milk, this marks a real advance in the protection of babies. Scientific understanding of the components of breast milk is incomplete, and formulas will probably never match the remarkable properties of human milk. They are, however, being improved all the time; they allow the mother freedom to work outside the home; and they enable the care of her child to be shared with other people.

Learning How to Handle Cholesterol

Breast milk is composed of lactose and fat. A question to which biologists have given much thought, though it is seldom raised in medical research, is whether the high contents of cholesterol and saturated fat in breast milk sets the way the baby handles cholesterol throughout its life. Is the amount of cholesterol in your blood a marker of the diet you received at this critical stage of your life, when your need for energy, previously met by carbohydrate and protein brought to you by the placenta, depended on a high-cholesterol, high-fat diet? In animals there is unequivocal evidence that interference with cholesterol handling during development permanently changes the way the body handles it. In humans slow growth during infancy is followed by altered cholesterol levels in the blood in adult life. These alterations in the balance of the different forms of cholesterol are of a kind that hastens hardening of the arteries in later life. This may be one reason why slow weight gain in infancy increases the risk of heart disease and stroke. Since cholesterol is regulated by the liver one suggestion, already referred to in Chapter 5, is that slow infant growth resets the liver during a sensitive period when it is learning how to handle cholesterol.

In the Hertfordshire studies, a group of mothers continued to breastfeed their children beyond the age of one year. These mothers tended to be in the poorer families, and they prolonged breastfeeding as a form of contraception. When their sons became adults they had higher cholesterol concentrations in their blood than other men, and higher death rates from coronary heart disease. Studies in baboons suggest that continued exposure to the thyroid hormone in mother's milk leads infants to reduce their own production of thyroid hormone—a response that persists and causes raised blood cholesterol levels in later life. Arguments about the optimal length of breastfeeding seldom take account of possible effects in later life.

WEANING

Weaning is defined as the process of expanding the diet to include food and drinks other than breast milk or infant formula. A baby can thrive on milk alone for the first four months after birth. During this time the gut is maturing and solid foods are not properly digested. In the last fifty years opinion about when to introduce solid food has changed. In the 1950s and 1960s introduction of solids as early as six weeks was popular. This is no longer recommended.

At some point in the infant's life the volume of milk that is needed to meet its increasing demands for energy becomes so great that it would be beyond an infant's capacity to drink it. The point at which this occurs will depend on the infant's size and speed of growth, and will therefore differ between one baby and another. In the US, babies fed on infant formula tend to be weaned earlier than those who are breast-fed. This may reflect different biological needs, as formula fed babies seem to need more energy than breast-fed babies.

In the mid-1970s there were concerns that early introduction of solids might be hazardous, leading to obesity. Introduction of solid foods before four months was discouraged, but mothers have paid little heed to this advice, and many babies receive some solid food before they reach this age. Family advice, a wish to have the baby sleep all night, or a desire to see it progressing to the next stage of development may lead mothers to begin weaning before four months. This may be inappropriate. Babies are born with a 'spitting up' reflex that persists for several months. The ability to move food around the mouth and chew does not readily develop before three to four months. Young infants do not digest solid food well and their kidneys may not be mature enough to handle the extra load which solid food imposes on them.

The World Health Organization recommends that all babies should be exclusively breast fed for six months. The reasoning behind this is that most of the serious infections that kill babies occur before six months of age, and breast feeding protects against them. In reality the length of time during which babies are fed on milk depends on the alternatives and on competing interests within the family. In Nepal women of the Tamang caste travel extensively up and down mountains to cultivate their crops and herd their animals. They are often away from home and have no alternative but to feed their infants on breast milk. Infants are fed whenever their demands coincide with the mother's ability to stop work. Breastfeeding continues for three years. The Tamang women have little choice other than to do this, as the alternative would be starvation. Across India, mothers have a wide range of weaning strategies to match their varying circumstances. In rural areas breastfeeding may be continued for two years, while office workers in the cities may discontinue long before six months. During weaning, the western infant can learn to enjoy a diversity of food offered at several meals a day, but for many infants in the world weaning is a harsh experience. In the towns of Tigrai, Ethiopia, half the infants receive only one daily meal of bread or porridge a day.

In humans and other mammals weaning may bring conflict between the interests of the mothers and the interests of the infants. In many communities across the world mothers who work outside the home have to give up breastfeeding early and change their infants to bottle feeding because their work benefits the family, whose interests are part of the equation that determines the infant's period of suckling. Age at weaning on to solid food is the result of a negotiation between each individual mother and her infant. It takes into account the biological needs of the mother, the infant and the rest of the family, and their wishes, whether cultural or individual. Inevitably there will be trade-offs. The age when a baby is weaned on to solid food is determined by a balance of interests, which may compete. There can be no universal prescription. What is the best age depends on the alternatives. What is right for one family is not right for another. What is best for one baby may not be best for another because each baby is different. The manufacturers of infant formulas are just beginning to move away from general recommendations and towards personalised regimes, tailored to fit the needs of each individual baby.

> *Age at weaning on to solid food is the result of a negotiation between each individual mother and her infant.*

WEANING NEGOTIATIONS IN OTHER MAMMALS

A new strategy to prevent chronic disease by improving the nutrition of girls and young women may need to be informed by the experiences of other animals. Much of what is known about growth in the womb comes from studies of sheep. All mammals have to wean their offspring. The weaning negotiations between the blue whale, the largest of mammals, and its calf involve hundreds of litres of milk. While being nursed the calf consumes more than 500 pints of milk each day and puts on 8 pounds in weight every hour. The whales breed in the winter in tropical or temperate waters and travel to polar waters to feed during the summer months. During the journey the calf cannot survive without the mother, but once the feeding grounds are reached the negotiation can begin. Mother and calf eventually part company, and the calf wanders off to fend for itself, having attained about 23 tons (20,900 kilograms) in weight and 52 feet (16 meters) in length after seven or eight months of suckling.

> *A new strategy to prevent chronic disease by improving the nutrition of girls and young women may need to be informed by the experiences of other animals.*

The weaning time of the blue whale is mainly determined by the pattern of its migrations through the oceans. The calf can only survive on its own once it has reached the feeding grounds. For other sea mammals local circumstances are more important. Stellar sea lions living off the Californian coast seldom suckle their young for more than a year before casting them off. To the north, in the harsher conditions of Alaska, they suckle them for two years. The age at weaning of bottlenose dolphins ranges from three to eight years. There seems to be no fixed age at weaning that is appropriate to all members of a species. This reinforces

> *This reinforces the view that the age for human weaning is an individual decision that depends on a balance of interests rather than on some over-riding biological imperative.*

the view that the age for human weaning is an individual decision that depends on a balance of interests rather than on some over-riding biological imperative.

Some animals anticipate weaning by conceiving their babies at particular times of the year. African bats conceive and give birth before the insects on which they feed are abundant. The completion of six weeks of suckling coincides with the ending of the rains and increasing abundance of insects. It takes the infant bats several weeks to learn how to catch and handle food efficiently, but through the mothers' foresight they do this at the time when there is most food available.

CONFLICT BETWEEN MOTHERS AND BABIES

The limited amount of food that is available to many mothers around the world may bring a conflict of interests between mother and baby. Elephant seals come ashore to breed on the island of South Georgia. Once on the beach the mothers do not eat. They nourish their pups from the reserves of protein and fat in their bodies. The proportion of the food reserves that is made available to the pups is critical to both mother and child. Mothers that expend a large proportion of their reserves on their pups may compromise their own survival to the next breeding season or reduce the number of offspring they have in the future. On the other hand, if their pups are born small and thin their chances of surviving to breeding age are reduced. The size of a pup is a compromise between the future reproductive success of the mother and the survival of the pup. Male pups are heavier at birth than females and the smallest elephant seal mothers only give birth to females: presumably they abort male pups. This may be an advantage if they are unable to raise a male pup to a viable size without jeopardising their own survival.

The theory of 'parent-child conflict' proposes that natural selection encourages babies to demand more resources from parents than parents are selected to give. Three sets of genes have different interests: the mother's genes, the baby's genes derived from the mother, and the baby's genes derived from the father. If the genes of any individual baby are permitted to make excessive demands on the mother it will, like the male pup in the young elephant seal, prejudice her ability to pass her genes on to future children. During evolution a baby's genes will have been selected to increase the transfer of food to it, from the mother, so that it can grow larger. Big babies are more likely to survive than small babies. A mother's genes will have been selected to limit transfer of food to the baby in order to protect the mother, and to ensure her survival and that of her other children, born and unborn. What is best for a baby need not be best for its mother, or so it seems.

The genes that the baby has derived from its father, however, have been selected to take more resources from the mother's tissues than the genes derived from the mother. The father's genes promote the baby's growth irrespective of the mother's well-being, for he can have more children by other mothers. The conflict between maternal and paternal genes over the nutritional demands that the fetus imposes on the mother may explain why genes derived from one parent can 'imprint', or over-ride, the expression of those derived from the other. An intriguing, though speculative theory suggests that preeclampsia and other diseases of pregnancy originate in the turmoil of this genetic conflict.

When adolescent girls become pregnant there is conflict between their need for food in order to continue to grow and the needs of their baby.

Beyond these fascinating genetic theories it is clear that in the distribution of food there is often conflict within a family. In times of famine Chinese peasants used to give their daughters away. When adolescent girls become pregnant there is conflict between their need for food in order to continue to grow and the needs of their baby. The blue petrel alternates long feeding trips out to sea with short feeding trips near the shore. Although the short trips increase the rate at which the chicks are fed, the father and mother lose weight. On long trips they feed themselves and restore their weight while the chicks have to wait longer for food. A human mother may wish to breastfeed her baby for six months, but be unable to do so if she is working away from home, and the income and well-being of herself and her family requires that this continues. This is a conflict rooted in our evolutionary past.

DEALING WITH FOOD SHORTAGES

In animals both mothers and fathers have strategies to meet food shortages. The aim is to reduce deaths among the offspring and maximise the fitness of the survivors. The red fox lives in Arctic Sweden where it feeds on voles. The numbers of voles fluctuate through the seasons and over three- to four-year cycles. The vixens mate in January or February, and when the spring comes in May they are already in late pregnancy or lactating. This doubles their food requirements, and the food supply becomes critical. Matters are so arranged, however, that the number of cubs they carry is appropriate to the abundance of voles in the area: the more abundant the voles, the more cubs are born. How is such a useful adaptation achieved?

The number of cubs is determined by the number of eggs released from the vixen's ovaries before mating. In mammals, food shortage reduces the number of eggs that are released, because it reduces the amount of a hormone, gonadotrophin, which is made in the pituitary gland and stimulates the ripening of follicles in the ovary. Because of the seasonal cycles the abundance of voles in the mating season, January to February, is not, however, closely related to the abundance in the spring when the cubs are born. Somehow when they mate the vixens respond, not to the amount of food they are eating at the time, but to the amount they predict will be available in the spring. It is in the interests of both the mother and her cubs that she does not carry more cubs than she can nourish during late pregnancy and lactation when she requires a lot of food. How, in January, does she predict the number of voles that will be around in May?

It might, of course, be inherited knowledge, like the salmon's knowledge of the routes and timetables which guide its wanderings through the oceans. But the seasonal fluctuation in vole numbers varies from year to year, and between one locality and the next. A plastic system operated by an environmental cue would seem a better option. It seems that the cue is the hormone levels in the voles. During the winter months voles only breed if their numbers are increasing. When they are not breeding they produce less gonadotrophin hormone. This hormone stimulates not only their ovaries but the ovaries of the vixens that eat them. Less stimulation to the vixen's ovaries results in fewer cubs

Another Arctic creature that preys on voles, the Tengmalm's Owl, has another form of anticipatory behaviour. During the upward fluctuation in the vole cycle the female owls produce the largest clutches of eggs and, through the night, the males fly back and forth feeding the females, and their offspring when they hatch. When the vole cycle is at its peak, however, and food is at its most abundant, the males lose interest, and deliver less food to the nest. After midnight they spend more time feeding themselves and resting. When they return to the nest they are less interested in defending it from pine martins that come to take the eggs. The explanation for this seemingly inappropriate behaviour seems to be that after the peak vole numbers may crash abruptly. Many offspring will die, and it may be advantageous for the parents to provide for a few well-fed owlets rather than many starving ones.

Human reproduction responds to food shortages at the time they occur, though because the human mother only carries one baby she has fewer options. In the Dutch famine there were more miscarriages and fewer boys were born. Surprisingly the girls who were in the womb at the time of the famine have had greater reproductive success, more children, than those conceived after the famine was over. For which, once again, there is no known explanation.

WEANING FOODS

Babies are usually ready to start on solid foods between the ages of four and six months, progressing over the weeks from puréed food to solids that they can pick up with their fingers. As teeth erupt, biting and chewing replace sucking. These feeding skills have to be acquired and pave the way for the successful introduction of solid foods. Porridge-type foods based on rice are common first weaning foods. Cereals (except wheat), fruit, vegetables and potatoes, are also used. General advice is that puréed fruit and vegetables should not be the sole first weaning foods, because they contain too little energy and fat. Yet mothers in Spain use puréed vegetables successfully by adding olive oil to increase their fat content.

Weaning is an opportunity to offer the baby a wide variety of foods, and introduce it to the range of textures and tastes that will form its diet through life. Common sense suggests that lifetime food preferences may be developed at this time, but there is a remarkable absence of knowledge about this, part of a wider ignorance of how early nutrition sets appetite. Breastfed babies may be better able to adjust to new foods

> *Weaning is an opportunity to offer the baby a wide variety of foods, and introduce it to the range of textures and tastes that will form its diet through life.*

> *Breastfed babies may be better able to adjust to new foods because mother's milk has a range of flavors and odors that are lacking from formula.*

> *Chewing improves the coordination of the mouth and tongue, which is important for the development of speech as well as eating skills.*

because mother's milk has a range of flavors and odors that are lacking from formula. After six months, the texture of the food needs to change gradually so that the child learns to chew better, whole food replacing puréed and mashed food. Chewing improves the coordination of the mouth and tongue, which is important for the development of speech as well as eating skills.

Recently a thousand mothers were asked their views on the choice of weaning foods; 95% considered a wide variety to be important. Disturbingly, over 80% thought that high-fiber, low-fat diets were also important. Although this view of an ideal infant diet was not always translated into action, it is a stark illustration of how traditional dietary practices have been distorted by single-issue enthusiasts, whether it is the healthy eating lobby extolling "fiber is good for you" or the 'anti-lobby' saying "butter kills".

In a recent study of six-month-old babies in Britain a nurse visited each home and interviewed the mother or the principal carer. The mother was asked about how the baby had been fed since birth and the previous day's food was recorded. The thousands of babies in the study were from families with a wide range of incomes, homes, ethnic backgrounds and lifestyles. The study illustrated problems shared by women across the western world.

One group of babies had already been completely weaned off milk and were drinking water, squash or diluted cow's milk. They were being under fed, as a baby requires energy from both food and milk for some months after weaning begins. Another group of babies was also being fast-tracked through the weaning process, but in a different way. They were being given foods such as toast and biscuits which, as they had no teeth, they could not chew. They too were being underfed. Other babies were being fed exclusively on jars of baby foods and formula: their diets lacked variety of texture and were expensive. Manufactured baby foods are designed to contribute to the immediate needs of a brief phase of life, weaning. They are an adjunct to the process of weaning onto family foods, but not a substitute.

Anemia is common in babies in the poorer areas of the US. At birth, the baby of even a well-nourished mother only has sufficient iron stores to carry it through the first six months. Breast milk is a poor source of iron and babies that have been exclusively breastfed commonly begin the second six months with low iron stores. Solid foods such as meat, fish, dark green vegetables, bread, and pulses (peas, beans and lentils) allow the infant to meet its needs for iron. Iron in meat and fish is more easily absorbed than iron contained in cereals and pulses

Anemia is common in babies in the poorer areas of the US. At birth, the baby of even a well-nourished mother only has sufficient iron stores to carry it through the first six months.

Meat, peas, beans, lentils and whole-wheat products are not only good sources of iron, but also provide zinc, a nutrient essential for child growth that is found in lesser amounts in refined cereal products. Children whose diets are deficient in zinc fail to grow. There is a strong lobby that advocates supplementing the diets of pregnant women in poor countries with zinc. Though it may seem an attractive option, the 'magic bullet' approach to improving the health of pregnant women and their children in the developing world has many opponents, and there may even be trade-offs. A recent study in Bangladesh showed that zinc supplementation led to poor mental development.

Current recommendations are that from the age of six months infants receiving breast milk as their main drink should be given supplements of vitamins A and D.

Current recommendations are that from the age of six months infants receiving breast milk as their main drink should be given supplements of vitamins A and D. Infants fed on formula do not need vitamin supplements, provided they consume more than one pint (500 ml) per day.

INDEPENDENCE

Biology demands that the child is set free from its dependence on the mother. Weaning is part of this journey.

Biology demands that the child is set free from its dependence on the mother. Weaning is part of this journey. It carries the infant from dependence on a high-fat diet to a varied adult diet in which most of the energy is supplied by carbohydrates. Even in western countries this seems for many babies to be a difficult journey. They risk being underfed, are offered monotonous diets and they may not learn to enjoy new foods. When an infant refuses food, spits it out, tips it over, puts its hand in it or throws it on the floor, it is taking part in a universal drama.

Infants quickly learn to try and get their own way and may reject savoury foods if they know that a sweet food, which they usually prefer, will eventually be given. It is a common observation that weaning behaviour, with a child getting its own way, rejecting savoury foods in favor of sweet foods, refusing to explore new foods, may continue through early childhood. It is as though weaning negotiations that should have ceased at the age of one are still in progress. Persistence of weaning behaviour long after weaning has ceased has varying manifestations. A child may successfully manipulate its own diet so that only pizza and burgers are offered. The child's continuing desire for fatty foods, possibly a legacy of its happy experiences of milk, may lead it, after victory over the mother, to a diet of fatty and sugary foods. The baby's liking for sweet food, and breast milk is remarkably sweet, may persist and transform into demands for sweets and confectionery.

The reluctance of a baby to abandon milk and experiment with other foods may lead to a childhood diet which is limited in variety with the child clinging to familiar and readily palatable foods.

> *The reluctance of a baby to abandon milk and experiment with other foods may lead to a childhood diet which is limited in variety…*

Unlike the Blue Whale, who abandons her child at a time when it can become fully independent, the weaning dialogue between the human mother and her baby is protracted, and at the end of it the child is still not independent of the mother. For our forbears, and for many women in the world today, the choices of weaning foods were and remain limited. Today western parents have new choices—dried baby foods, fortified foods, organic foods and baby food in jars and cans. They can buy their toddlers food shaped like animals or letters of the alphabet, food with toys, cartoon characters made from pasta or teddy bears made from crisps. These are diversions: the core of successful weaning remains unchanged. Over a period, food gradually replaces milk so that by one year it comprises most of the diet. Though the infants may initially resist, they have an instinct to experiment with an increasing variety of food of different textures and tastes. Biologically they cannot remain forever dependent on the mother, and must set themselves free. For many babies weaning is preceded by separation, when breastfeeding ceases and this private dialogue between mother and baby is discontinued. Finally, the child reaches the fourth phase of its changing relationship with its mother. In the womb, it lives off her body and what goes into her mouth: after birth, it lives off her breast milk: then it lives off weaning food: finally it lives off family food.

SUMMARY

Infancy lasts from birth to two years of age. People grow more rapidly during this time than they do at any later age. Almost one quarter of the energy available to an infant is used for growth. Two large organs, the brain and the liver, together with the immune system, remain plastic for some years after birth and can still be permanently changed. Infants who grow slowly tend to achieve less at school and during their working lives and are at increased risk of high blood pressure, heart disease, stroke and diabetes in later life. Through their lives their livers handle cholesterol, which they have received in large amounts in breast milk, in a way that promotes hardening of the arteries.

After birth bacteria colonise the baby's intestines. This process begins moments before birth when the baby, who has never encountered bacteria, enters its mother's vagina. There, for the first time, it meets the bacteria which will form the flora of its intestines for the rest of its life, a stable ecosystem that fuels the recycling plant in the colon, and synthesises new foods from the body's waste.

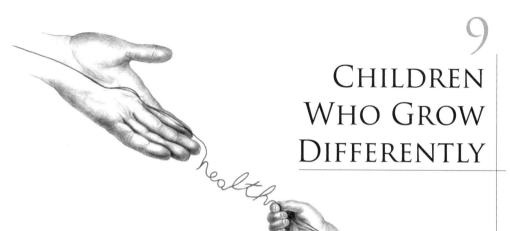

9

CHILDREN
WHO GROW
DIFFERENTLY

WE ARE UNIQUE AMONG ANIMALS. We walk on two legs and have large brains. We can breed in any season, in any climate. But though our growth is different from that of other animals, it is governed by the same processes. It responds to our surroundings through a blueprint laid down in our distant evolutionary past.

HOW CHILDREN GROW

After infancy, the first two years after birth, the rate of growth slows. An infant uses a quarter of its energy for growth whereas a two-year old uses only 6 percent. From two years until puberty a child grows at a relatively constant rate of around 2 inches in height per year. Although growth rates may be constant from year to year, new research shows that it is episodic from day to day. Over a few days a child ceases to grow but its appetite increases and it eats more. During the following few days it grows.

The growth of most organs follows that of the body as a whole. The brain is an exception: it grows in advance of the body. By around 7 years the head has reached about 80% of its final size, whereas length is only 65% of final height. After 7 years there is a small spurt in the rate of the body's growth that heralds the onset of puberty, when the adolescent growth spurt occurs. Whereas girls increase the amount of fat after puberty boys increase their muscle mass and may even lose fat.

A growing child needs energy for four main activities: staying alive, growing, keeping warm and moving. The first of these requires the most energy. The extent of this requirement, known as the basal metabolic rate, is mainly determined by four organs, the brain, liver, heart and kidney. These organs use 65 percent of the energy needed to stay alive. Peoples different metabolic rates may determine why, in periods of starvation, some people perish while others survive.

> *A growing child needs energy for four main activities: staying alive, growing, keeping warm and moving.*

HEIGHT IS NOT JUST GENETIC

Mankind has known for thousands of years that undernutrition reduces the growth of animals: the scientific literature is enormous. Surprisingly, the link between poor nutrition and poor growth in humans only became accepted relatively recently. Until the last century, in both America and Europe, there was a strong 'hereditarian' school of thought. Its adherents believed that height was inherited because people's heights were generally related to those of their parents. In arguments that resonate with those we hear today, maintaining that our health is primarily determined by our genetic inheritance, the hereditarians proposed that inheritance was the main determinant of human form and function. Impoverished American children living in city slums or on poor farms were stunted, thin, and weak because they came from genetically inferior stock. Therefore there was no compelling reason to improve their lot. Rather, weakling infants and children should be allowed to perish, in order to maintain the physical quality of the nation.

In the US hereditarians believed that physically inferior people from Southern and Eastern Europe, who were immigrating into America in large numbers, would bring about the physical deterioration of the American people, and their inter-marriage with Anglo-Saxons would weaken the stock for many generations. Franz Boas, an anthropologist, championed the anti-hereditarian cause. In a famous study in New York, Boas demonstrated that immigrant children who were born in America were taller and heavier than their parents had been at the same age, and differently shaped as well. Boas ascribed this to the better nutrition and health of children in America. His conclusion that the environment has a major influence on growth is now generally accepted, but at the time it collided with the strongly held view that human types and races are fixed by inheritance. Notwithstanding his correct scientific conclusion, the hereditarians campaigned successfully for a reduction in migration quotas from southern and eastern Europe.

> *In a famous study in New York, Boas demonstrated that immigrant children who were born in America were taller and heavier than their parents had been at the same age, and differently shaped as well.*

Boas continued to fight the idea that immigrants from poor countries were genetically destined to remain inferior for many generations. He went on to study their tempo of growth. The importance of this had already been proposed by the mathematician, naturalist and Greek scholar, D'Arcy Thompson. His book *"On Growth and Form"*, published in 1917 is still read today: "To say that children of a given age vary in the rate at which they are growing would seem to be a more fundamental statement than that they vary in the size to which they have grown."

The smaller body size of people who grow up in hardship is more the result of individual responses during one lifetime than the effects of genes selected across many generations. Even the small size of pygmies is not linked to any known genes. In parts of Africa, as their diets improve pygmies are now growing taller! The plasticity of our growth allows us to adapt rapidly to changing circumstances brought by migration, famine and war. It has given us an advantage we would not have if we developed along a rigid genetic plan. It allows us to inhabit the arctic, savannah, desert and tropical rain forest.

Human growth responds to adverse conditions in various ways.

Human growth responds to adverse conditions in various ways. Slowing of growth is one response; another is delay in the final maturation of the skeleton, allowing growth to continue for longer; and a third is to delay sexual maturation, the onset of puberty, and thereby delay the adolescent growth spurt.

Whereas in the US young boys and girls in affluent families achieve their final heights at around 21 years and 18 years of age respectively, children in malnourished communities continue their growth for longer. Growth can continue until around 25 years of age, allowing more time for those whose growth has been slowed to catch up. In the European armies of the 19th century the young officers were much taller than new recruits. They had grown up in better circumstances. In their early 20s, however, the soldiers caught up. They were still growing while the officers' growth had ceased.

It is usually better for a female animal to delay reproduction until she is fully grown because her offspring are more likely to survive. If, however, young females are under threat from their environment, early sexual maturation reduces the risk of death before reproduction. Humans mature sexually before their growth is complete. This has the disadvantage that, when an adolescent girl becomes pregnant, mother and baby may compete for resources for growth, a common occurrence in Asia today. The mother's needs take precedence over the baby's, and food supplements benefit her growth but not that of her baby.

The timing of sexual maturation responds to the conditions of an individual's life. Over the past century the age of onset of menstruation, menarche, among Finnish girls has fallen from 17 to 13 years of age. More food and better living conditions have permitted both more rapid growth and earlier sexual maturation. Once a girl has menstruated her growth is almost complete. The average girl grows only about 2 inches (6 cm) after menarche. The delayed onset of sexual maturation in European girls in the past allowed them to continue to grow for a longer period.

A group of young girls living in an orphanage in India were adopted by Swedish families and went to live in Sweden. On arrival, they were thin and stunted, but with better food and living conditions their weights and heights increased rapidly. For reasons that are little understood, this rapid growth induced early sexual maturation. The Indian girls began to menstruate at an average age of 11½ years, well before the Swedish girls among whom they lived. Having begun to menstruate, their growth ceased. To the dismay of their adoptive parents they ended up no taller than the girls left behind in the orphanages. Biology sometimes mocks good intentions. It is an irony that in America better childcare and living conditions have prolonged life but shortened childhood!

It is an irony that in America better childcare and living conditions have prolonged life but shortened childhood!

Through childhood, tall children tend to remain taller than other children, while short children tend to remain shorter. It is as if body size is on railroad tracks. At some age around two years, growth

At some age around two years, growth rates become 'set' by the internal environment and are less sensitive to the day-to-day supply of food. Until then food has commanded the rate of growth. Now the rate of growth commands the need for food.

rates become 'set' by the internal environment and are less sensitive to the day-to-day supply of food. Until then food has commanded the rate of growth. Now the rate of growth commands the need for food. Excess food will not lead to more growth, but to fatness. The external environment still influences growth rates in childhood, but the child's initial response to adversity is to try and maintain its growth, to stay in its track.

THE HORMONES THAT CONTROL GROWTH

Growth involves the division of cells and their expansion, and the accumulation of substances between cells such as the minerals in bone. The proliferation of cells has to be finely controlled so that the final number of cells in each organ is adequate to meet the demands imposed both by other organs within the body and by the external environment. Growth depends on adequate nutrition but also on hormones, which coordinate growth in different parts of the body.

Insulin regulates growth before birth and continues to do so until some point around one year of age when a new messenger, 'growth hormone', takes over. This heralds the second of three phases of human growth after birth. The first, infancy, is a continuation of growth in the womb; the second is childhood; and the third pubertal. At puberty, the sex hormones, testosterone and estrogen, take on an important role in regulating growth.

Because childhood growth is controlled by hormones whose release is controlled by the brain, it is possible to understand how psychological stress may impair growth despite adequate nutrition.

Among German children who were orphaned during the second war, those placed in an orphanage with a harsh punitive regime put on less weight than those in an orphanage with a gentler regime, despite having an identical diet. Few mothers would quarrel with the idea that happy children grow better.

A difficulty in understanding differences in body size between one child and another is that events at one point in time can have 'down-stream' effects, which change growth several years later. In the US, girls who grow up in less affluent homes tend to have less muscle and bone but more fat. Examination of a national sample showed that this was already evident at birth but became increasingly apparent up to the age of seven. We do not know whether this amplification after birth is a consequence of poor living conditions or whether it is pre-determined by poor muscle development in the womb.

A difficulty in understanding differences in body size between one child and another is that events at one point in time can have 'down-stream' effects, which change growth several years later.

THE GROWTH OF CHILDREN WHO LATER DEVELOP CHRONIC DISEASE

Johan Eriksson, a Finnish physician, discovered what may prove to be the world's most detailed set of records of the growth, illnesses and living conditions of a large group of men and women now approaching old age. From early in the last century the size of all babies born in the two maternity hospitals in Helsinki, Finland, was measured in detail. As described in Chapter 3 child welfare clinics were established in the city in 1934 and recorded growth between birth and school age. At school the children's growth continued to be recorded by two doctors who visited each school in the city every 6 months. The growth records of more than 13,000 people born during 1934 to 1944 have been computerized. For each person there are on average 18 measurements of height and weight from birth to eleven years of age!

Finland has a unique personal identification number for each of its citizens. For the purposes of research, this number can be used to determine whether a person is alive or dead, what they died of, whether they have ever been admitted to hospital, and if so with what illness, and whether they are taking medicines for chronic disease. By studying the 13,000 people, it has been possible to see, for the first time, whether people who developed stroke, coronary heart disease and diabetes grew differently when they were children.

They did! The children who suffered from a stroke in their later lives were short at birth and grew slowly during infancy, so that at two years of age they were short and thin. After that they remained small. Their slow growth during infancy was not related to the living conditions into which they were born. As Chapter 7 described stroke has its origins in the mother's nutrition since she was a girl. The children who later developed heart disease had low birthweight and low placental weight and they too put on weight slowly during infancy. Their slow infant growth was partly the result of poor living conditions, with recurrent minor infections. At two years of age they were thin. After that age, however, they began to put on weight at a greater rate than other children. This was not matched by similar rapid growth in height, so that their weights in relation to their heights, their body mass indices, increased. It was as though the children, having been thin, tried to 'catch-up' with the others.

The path of growth of children who went on to receive treatment for diabetes was initially similar to that of children who developed heart disease. Small size at birth was followed by slow growth up to the age of two years. After this they put on weight rapidly;

but unlike the children who later developed heart disease, whose weight caught up with the average for all the children, those who later developed diabetes not only caught up but continued to gaining weight rapidly. It was as though, having fallen behind in a race, they not only caught up with the pack but raced through it to take the lead.

In a class of eleven year old schoolchildren in Helsinki at that time three groups of children were at risk of developing chronic disease in later life. In their later lives a group of short, thin children had strokes, a group of short children of average fatness had heart disease and a group of slightly overweight children went on to develop diabetes. Their body size alone did not distinguish these children. They would not have stood out from other children in the class. What distinguished them was the path of growth by which they had attained their body size, a path characterised by slow growth in the womb and during the first two years after birth sometimes followed by rapid 'catch-up' or 'compensatory' weight gain thereafter. Most children at risk of chronic disease are invisible unless their growth has been recorded serially from birth. Every French child has such a record. Almost no American children do. In recent years a new group of children has joined the three groups of children in the Helsinki classrooms. These are children who are already obese, may have been obese at birth, and are destined to develop diabetes at an early age, even in childhood. Obesity represents another form of malnutrition, in which insufficiency is replaced by unbalanced and monotonous excess.

In their later lives a group of short, thin children had strokes, a group of short children of average fatness had heart disease and a group of slightly over-weight children went on to develop diabetes.

RAPID WEIGHT GAIN IN CHILDHOOD

In general, we view growth as good. We are glad when our children grow. There must, however, be 'costs' and trade-offs attached to fast growth. The rule for living things seems to be that if energy is allocated to rapid growth, the allocation to some other activity or activities must be reduced. People who go fishing know that the size of fish varies according to local conditions. In some small streams, trout never weigh more than 2 ounces. In nearby lakes they can be a hundred times larger. If rapid growth has costs, why do the trout in the lake grow so large? The broad answer must be that the costs must be worth paying. If small size makes an animal more vulnerable to predators, or if it needs to reach a certain body size in order to survive the winter, the advantages of rapid growth will offset the costs.

It is a common observation that after a child's growth has slowed because of illness it will, on recovery, 'catch up' so that the child returns to the size it would have been had it not become ill. The ability to mount 'compensatory growth' is common in animals. Farmers are familiar with it: they know that after an inclement season young animals that have been undernourished recover and reach normal mature heights and weights. This ability to compensate for undernutrition may be essential for animals, which in their wild state are often subjected to periods of near starvation. Compensatory growth is driven by large increases in appetite. In some circumstances this increased appetite may persist after body size has been restored. Is the rapid and sustained weight gain of children who were thin at two years of age and who later develop diabetes the result of a persisting increase in appetite? Once again we do not know.

Slowing of growth during infancy or childhood can lead to immediate compensatory growth when adequate nutrition is restored. If shortage of food persists, however, compensation may be delayed until adolescence. After the importation of slaves from Africa was abolished in 1807, all slaves transported by sea from one port in the US to another had to have their names, ages, sex and heights recorded on the ship's manifest. Fifty thousand such records have recently been analysed. The slave children were stunted in comparison with modern children. At around 15 years of age, however, they began to grow rapidly so that they even exceeded the average height of Americans today. This rapid growth coincided with their being better fed, because they had reached an age when they were able to do adult physical work.

THE COSTS OF RAPID WEIGHT GAIN IN CHILDHOOD

Rapid growth has a surprising range of costs in animals. We are beginning to understand the costs in children. Some of them are deferred until later life. Chapter 5 described how babies with low birthweight have fewer functioning units, nephrons, in the kidney. If during childhood they have compensatory weight gain, the larger sized body will impose a greater workload on each nephron. The blood flow through each will be greater than it would otherwise have been. This will not have immediate consequences, but in later life it will hasten the death of nephrons that accompanies aging, leading to raised blood pressure.

When young undernourished cattle restore their body weights by compensatory growth, the composition of their bodies is not the same as if they had not been undernourished. They will have less muscle, but more fat. There seems to be a similar phenomenon in humans. Babies who grow slowly before birth and during infancy have less muscle, because this is the critical period for muscle growth. After around one year of age no new muscle can be made, though existing muscle can enlarge. Rapid weight gain after the age of two years will increase the amount of fat and lead to an adult body with a high proportion of fat to muscle. This increases the body's resistance to insulin, and is linked to both heart disease and diabetes.

Much more is known about the costs of rapid growth in animals then is known in humans. Human research is at its beginnings because we have only recently recognized the importance of the topic.

Much more is known about the costs of rapid growth in animals then is known in humans. Human research is at its beginnings because we have only recently recognized the importance of the topic. In farm animals and fish rapid growth increases susceptibility to infections, reduces the quality of tissues such as bone and shortens lifespan. For this reason farmers do not force the growth of young animals as much as modern technology could allow them to. Animals give us insights into processes that may be important to humans.

The life of the salmon opens up interesting new possibilities for the links between growth and heart disease. Salmon develop blockages in the arteries of their heart walls, the coronary arteries, which are similar to those that cause heart disease and death in humans. These blockages accumulate slowly as the young salmon grow in the rivers in which they were born. When they reach the sea, however, the numbers and severity of the blockages increase rapidly. By the time they are sexually mature, at around 4 years of age, 95% of them have blockages.

The explanation seems to lie in the change of diet once they reach the sea. While young salmon are in their nursery streams they live on the sparse proteins they are able to obtain from small aquatic insects, and they grow slowly. Once at sea, however, they eat fish, rich in fat, and grow faster. We do not know why this change of diet accelerates the blockage of their coronary arteries, but this story of the poor diet in the rivers followed by the high fat diet at sea, resonates remarkably with the story of the person who develops heart disease—a poor diet in the womb and during infancy followed by a high fat diet in childhood.

REDUCED LIFESPAN

We do not know to what extent the salmon's rapid growth shortens its life span. Other animals provide evidence on this. The fast-growing lizards in the meadows of Brittany lead shorter lives than the slow-growing lizards in the mountains of southern France. The caterpillars of speckled wood butterflies living in the sunny island of Madeira grow slowly, because the butterflies can reproduce all the year round, so there is no haste to grow large, become a pupa and emerge as an adult. Speckled wood butterflies in colder places can only reproduce in the summer. The caterpillars grow fast and they lead shorter lives. Allocating more resources to growth reduces the allocation to functions such as body maintenance and repair.

This can be shown experimentally. Rats that were undernourished in the womb and remained undernourished after they were born, lived for longer than those who were undernourished in the womb but given a better diet after birth. The lives of the latter were shortened by the human equivalent of 20 years. High food intake after birth and rapid compensatory growth seem to lead to a short life.

ALTERED ORGAN SIZE

Experiments with piglets and lambs have shown that the size of different organs can be manipulated by different kinds of feeding. Three groups of pigs were fed in different ways; but all ended up with the same body weight. The weights of their livers were markedly different. The group that had been under nourished early on and then well fed had larger livers than the group that had been adequately fed throughout. Little is known about how early growth affects organ size in humans. Studies carried out almost a century ago showed that people in India, Africa and Europe, whose paths of childhood growth are very different, differ in the relative sizes of their organs. Though this was of only passing interest to anthropologists at the time, it could prove important to the themes of this book.

WEAKENED BONES

Slow growth reduces the requirement for food and allows longer intervals between feeding. It also enables nutrients to be used more efficiently. Rapid growth may reduce the quality of the body's tissues. The time required to grow bone is one of the factors that constrain the speed of growth. Specialized bone cells, called osteoblasts, make a fibrous scaffolding around which are deposited the calcium salts that make the bone hard. This 'mineralization' of each new piece of bone takes around 10 days.

Young cranes need to make a lot of bone because they have long legs. One species, the Sand Hill Crane, is endangered and a group of them were taken to the Wildlife Research Center in Florida. No-one really knew what an ideal diet was for a young crane, and so they were fed generously with a high-protein diet. They grew rapidly, but suddenly, around three weeks after hatching, their legs began to twist and bend and the joints dislocated. Tests showed that there was sufficient calcium and phosphorous in their diets: examination of their bones showed no disease. Instead, it seemed that they had been over-fed: the bones had grown faster than the crystals could form, so that they were weakened. The Sand Hill Crane belongs to an assortment of animals, which include horses, poultry and Great Danes, which have the capacity to grow fast but reduce the quality of their bones in doing so.

Many elderly people fracture their hips, spines or wrists because they suffer from osteoporosis, thin bones. Current ideas about the causes of osteoporosis are focussed on adult lifestyles, on smoking, lack of exercise, diets lacking calcium, and, of course, on genes. But just as with heart disease, the idea that thin bones are retribution for bad habits goes only a small way to explaining why one person fractures their hip or spine while another does not. Recent research has shown that elderly people who fracture their hips grew differently to other people as children. Osteoporosis is another disease that is initiated through slow growth in early life followed by more rapid growth. If bones grow at a rate that is too fast to allow proper mineralization, the loss of minerals that comes inevitably with old age will bring weak bones, fracture and disability.

Recent research has shown that elderly people who fracture their hips grew differently to other people as children.

Rapid growth not only weakens bones through poor mineralization, but it may alter their mechanical properties in other ways. Weakened bones are more likely to deform if they have to bear heavy weights. Modern farm animals reach enormous weights, which put a strain on their bones. In pigs this may cause the upper end of the thigh bone to deform at the hip joint. When pigs grow fast under the artificial conditions of modern farming, the growth of the legs is unable to keep up with the growth of the trunk and as a result, the legs carry an excessive mechanical load. This leads to deformity around the hip—which may be relevant to humans in whom hip fractures are the most serious complication of osteoporosis.

Difficulties in combining rapid growth and a strong skeleton are shared by many animals. Snails make a skeleton that surrounds them rather than being within them. Periwinkle snails are abundant on the shores of New England. Their shape differs widely: some are round while others are conical, and there are all shapes in between. Inevitably this has been labelled as genetic variation, the result of natural selection; but a closer look shows that the conical snails live in places that are crowded with many periwinkles, while the round ones live more solitarily. Like other animals, it takes time for a snail to make a skeleton because there is a fixed rate at which calcium salts can be deposited. In less-crowded places there is more food and each snail grows faster. Given that the speed at which a shell can be made to cover the body is limited, a round shell is made because it allows more body to be accommodated than a conical one. The cost of a round shell, however, is that it is thinner and the periwinkle is more vulnerable to the dog whelks, star fish and crabs which prey upon it.

OTHER COSTS OF RAPID GROWTH

The experience of the orphaned Indian girls provides a dramatic demonstration that compensatory growth in children may be accompanied by profound disturbances in physiology. It was hoped that the better food and care they received in Sweden would make them into taller, sturdier adults. Instead, they matured sexually at such a young age that some doctors thought the girls must have tumors producing sex hormones. There seemed no biological gain from this. Rather, they completed growth early and ended up no taller than they would have been if they had remained in India.

A biologist once asked, "Why are mice the size they are?" There seems no mechanical reason why they should not be larger. Becoming larger must therefore have costs. Though larger mice will tend to have more offspring, perhaps they are more likely to fall prey to the many animals for which a mouse is food. This can now be put to the test because genetic engineering has produced "super mice". They make a hundred times more growth hormone than their brothers and sisters, grow twice as fast and become twice as large. But they sleep for twice as long and avoid any activity, even the grooming of their fur. The energy they have to allocate to growth leads to a crisis, with insufficient energy remaining for movement and normal behaviour.

When an animal grows rapidly, the symmetry of its body may be sacrificed. Some parts of the body are naturally asymmetrical: the human heart is on the left; male fiddler crabs have two claws, a small one for eating with and a large one for waving rhythmically at female fiddler crabs during courtship. But much of the body's function depends on symmetry: legs of the same length, wings of the same size. Symmetry may also be important for the selection of mates. Beautiful human faces tend to be symmetrical. Among those species of birds in which the males have exaggerated plumage for use in courtship rituals, the females seem to prefer those with symmetrical plumage. Symmetry may have importance beyond the choice of mates. Symmetrical, hence more attractive, juveniles may get more food from their parents. More attractive adults may have better social relations with other adults.

The growth of living things may be restrained so that the benefits of having a large body are not outweighed by the costs of acquiring it. Growth does not proceed with all possible speed until some mechanical constraint is reached and the body can grow no faster.

The growth of living things may be restrained so that the benefits of having a large body are not outweighed by the costs of acquiring it.

MONITORING CHILDREN'S GROWTH

Since the days when Boas was studying immigrant children in New York, concerns about growth in height in the US have largely been resolved. The stunted children in slums and poor farms have mostly disappeared. But in human biology change brings new challenges.

...in human biology change brings new challenges.

Improved nutrition has shortened childhood. It has also brought obesity. In old movies and newsreels, overweight people are strikingly absent. Today

Improved nutrition has shortened childhood. It has also brought obesity.

increasing numbers of children are attaining levels of overweight which were previously unknown. In the same way as for adults a child's fatness is usually measured by its body mass index. Chart 1 enables this to be calculated for any child whose weight and height are known. A high body mass index indicates a fatter child, though the index is not a direct measure of fat and a child may have a high body mass index because it is exceptionally muscular. The waist circumference provides an additional check because fat children generally have large waists while muscular children do not.

Charts 2 and 3 show the changes in body mass index of boys and girls as they grow. They allow the body mass index of a child to be related to that of other children of the same age. This relative body mass is expressed as 'centiles', which range from 1, the thinnest children, to 100, the fattest. A child of average fatness is therefore on the 50th centile. As they grow, children tend to stay on the same centile lines. Children who fail to thrive tend to become thin before their growth in height slows. They therefore cross centile lines for body mass index downwards before crossing those for height. In some children who fail to thrive a clinical illness is discovered. In others, the cause may be feeding problems or psychological difficulties. A child that is undernourished because of feeding or behavioural problems may show no signs of being hungry or be eager to feed when food is offered. Children who consume snacks and large volumes of dilute sweetened juices frequently have poor appetites for more nutritious foods.

As they grow, children tend to stay on the same centile lines.

Children who consume snacks and large volumes of dilute sweetened juices frequently have poor appetites for more nutritious foods.

Charts 2 and 3 are based on American children and would be inappropriate in many other countries, and may also be inappropriate for immigrants. They show that body mass index changes as children grow older. Between birth and one year babies get fatter and their body mass indices rise sharply. After that age, as the child grows taller, but does not continue to require large fat stores, the body mass index falls. At around six years of age the body mass index begins to rise again, the so called 'adiposity rebound'. The timing of the adiposity rebound is critically important to the later development of obesity and diabetes. Inspection of Charts 2 and 3 shows that among children who remained thin, having the lowest body mass indices throughout childhood, the body mass index did not begin to rise until around eight years. Among children with the highest body mass indices the rebound occurred at around four years. Adiposity rebound at an early age is now known to predict obesity and diabetes in adult life. It gives us a new framework within which to monitor children's fatness, and it can help to identify those who will become diseased long before they do.

> *At around six years of age the body mass index begins to rise again, the so called 'adiposity rebound'. The timing of the adiposity rebound is critically important to the later development of obesity and diabetes.*

In the past decade it seemed a reasonable policy to try to lower the levels of fatness by improving the diets and increasing the physical activity of schoolchildren. Attempts to do this on a large scale have been extremely disappointing. The strategy is also flawed conceptually. From studies in which children have been followed up from infancy we know that adult obesity begins before school age. Some children are fat as infants and remain fat through childhood and into adolescence. They are at risk of being obese adults and some will develop diabetes. The Helsinki study has shown that there is a second group of children who are at increased risk of diabetes.

> *...adult obesity begins before school age.*

Until recently if a group of physicians was asked to identify which among a group of two-year old children were destined to develop diabetes in later life, they would have replied that it was the fattest ones. They would have been wrong. The Helsinki study has shown that the most dangerous path of growth begins with thinness. For reasons which we do not understand low weight gain during infancy, leading to thinness at two years, triggers an early adiposity rebound. When children first go to school those at most risk of later diabetes may not be the fattest but those who, having been thin at two years, have not yet reached even average levels of fatness. They are, however, the boys and girls who are putting on weight most rapidly, crossing centiles of body mass index upwards. This has a major effect on their risk of developing diabetes. If each of the Helsinki children had weighed more than 8 pounds at birth, and had remained in his or her track of body mass index between the ages of two and eleven years, the number of adults with diabetes would have been halved.

When children first go to school those at most risk of later diabetes may not be the fattest but those who, having been thin at two years, have not yet reached even average levels of fatness.

This shows the importance of measuring children's body mass indices at intervals from two years onwards. This will identify those who are gaining fat rapidly, crossing centiles of body mass index upwards. At present we use centile charts to relate the fatness of a child to that of other children of the same age. If the child is average or below, we are reassured. We should not be. It is not the fatness at any particular age that is the focus of concern; it is the rate of increase in a child's fatness. A child's size must be judged by the path of growth that brought it to that size, rather than by its size in relation to that of the other children around it.

It is not the fatness at any particular age that is the focus of concern; it is the rate of increase in a child's fatness.

PREVENTING AN EARLY ADIPOSITY REBOUND

What can be done if a child's body mass index begins to increase at four or five years of age? Although the precise causes of rapid childhood weight gain are widely debated, two culprits are universally acknowledged, snacking between meals and lack of physical exercise. Production and promotion of a completely new range of easily stored, ready-to-eat snacks, often high in sugar and fat, has been a major change in the American diet over the past 20 years. Children with weight problems often have undisciplined eating habits.

The decline in physical activity among American children is recognized as a major influence in the obesity epidemic. One of the strongest predictors of childhood obesity is the presence of a television in the child's bedroom! Increasingly, parents are afraid to allow their children to walk to school or roam the streets and footpaths. Structured physical recreation in schools and clubs has become the alternative way to maintain adequate levels of physical activity. In monkey colonies given access to unlimited food, the development of obesity in the young was unrelated to how much food each of them ate. Rather it depended on the amount of exercise, which was measured by an accelerometer, worn by each animal. Patterns of exercise varied widely between monkeys and for any individual were relatively constant from day to day. What establishes patterns of activity in infants and young children is unknown.

> *One of the strongest predictors of childhood obesity is the presence of a television in the child's bedroom!*

SUMMARY

The growth of living things does not proceed with all possible speed until some mechanical constraint is reached and they can grow no faster. Rather growth is optimized, limited so that the benefits of larger body size are not outweighed by costs. At some age around two years a child's rate of growth becomes 'set' by the internal environment and is less sensitive to the day-to-day supply of food. Until then food has commanded the rate of growth. Now the rate of growth commands the need for food. Excess food will not lead to more growth, but to fatness.

People who develop chronic diseases grow differently as children. A large group of children born in Helsinki, Finland, has been followed up for 65 years. At eleven years of age those who suffered strokes in later life were short and thin; those who developed heart disease were short and of average fatness; while those who developed diabetes were overweight. These children would not have stood out from other children in the class. What distinguished them was the path of growth by which they had attained their body size. This path was characterised by slow growth in the womb and during the first two years after birth followed, in some children, by rapid 'compensatory' weight gain. This path of growth leads to a high proportion of fat to muscle in the body, which is known to predispose to heart disease and diabetes. Children should have their growth recorded, as is done routinely in some European countries.

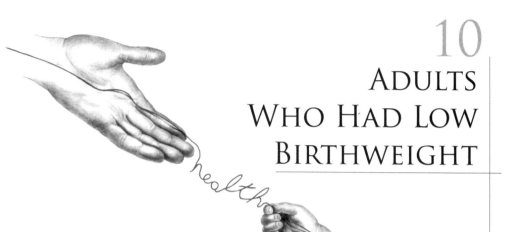

10
ADULTS WHO HAD LOW BIRTHWEIGHT

PEOPLE WHO HAD LOW BIRTH WEIGHT AGE MORE RAPIDLY

The western lifestyle has brought heart disease, diabetes and obesity but it has also brought a remarkable increase in the number of years we live. In the past hundred years the average lifespan in the US has increased from forty-nine to seventy-six years. We do not know why. Simple explanations like better food, better hygiene, better medical care, leave unexplained why people in Japan live longer than people in the US, or why, within the US, there is such a wide variation in lifespan.

Early pointers to the importance of the first few years of life in determining lifespan were calculations showing that, within western countries, each generation has lower death rates than the previous one at every age from birth to old age. It is as though from its earliest beginnings the vitality of each succeeding generation is enhanced beyond that of the generation that precedes it. Not only do a greater proportion of people attain eighty, ninety, even a hundred years of age but they reach these ages in better health: they are fitter and more mentally active than ever before. They are aging more slowly, so that at any given age they are biologically younger than previous generations. 75 years of age today is biologically the same as 65 years in the past. Within western countries, the places where people have the longest life expectancy are the places where people are not only healthier but are biologically younger. Evidence of this is all around us. The most casual observation shows that older people in more affluent, healthier places have smoother complexions, because they have more elastic skin, one of the biological markers of slower aging. In Scotland, old people in Edinburgh, the wealthy capital city, are four years biologically younger than people of the same age in nearby Glasgow, a historically poor city of slums and shipyards.

Within western countries, the places where people have the longest life expectancy are the places where people are not only healthier but are biologically younger.

The poor have shorter lives, another aspect of the poverty paradox which first directed attention to the importance of conditions in early life for lifetime health. Aging is inevitable, but the rate at which we age is determined by the conditions of our lives. The realisation that different paths of early growth and development make people more or less vulnerable to aging processes is new; and at this time we only see the picture in outline. It is clear, however, that low birthweight in a baby born at term is a simple and available marker of a path of development that is sub-optimal and makes a person vulnerable to the stresses of later life. There are two different challenges in middle and old age. One is to slow the rate of biological aging: the other is to prevent age-related diseases, importantly heart disease, stroke, diabetes and osteoporosis. The two challenges are linked but the second is not an inevitable consequence of the first.

Aging is inevitable, but the rate at which we age is determined by the conditions of our lives.

There are two different challenges in middle and old age. One is to slow the rate of biological aging: the other is to prevent age-related diseases.

WHAT IS HEALTH?

The World Health Organization defines health as "complete physical, mental and social well-being, not merely the absence of disease." Much of well-being is outside the influence of doctors. It is more than having a low blood pressure and cholesterol, taking exercise and remaining slim. It has a number of components, physical, mental, material and social among which the last three may be more important than the first. The components are related to each other and all are related to lifespan. Innumerable surveys have shown that elderly people who are inactive, failing mentally, impoverished and without social support have shorter lives.

WHY PEOPLE WHO HAD LOW BIRTHWEIGHT HAVE SHORTER LIVES

People differ in their inner environments, in the settings within their bodies by which they maintain an internal constancy. Some people need more sleep than others. Some people react more calmly to the ups and downs of life than others. These internal 'homeostatic' settings are established through our experience of the outside world as a baby, infant and young child. Once established, internal constancy has to be maintained in the face of assaults from the outside world, and failure to maintain constancy leads to disease—high blood pressure, high blood sugar, thin bones. People who had low birthweight have more fragile 'homeostatic' settings that are more readily perturbed by the outside world. They readily develop diabetes if they overeat and become obese. They are prone to high blood pressure if they become stressed.

People who had low birthweight have more fragile 'homeostatic' settings that are more readily perturbed by the outside world.

As far as we know, people who had low birthweight cannot change their internal settings. The option available to them is therefore to reduce the challenge to these settings. Their bodies need protection from the outside world, from excesses of lifestyle. "Low birth weight" is an abbreviation for "birthweight towards the lower end of the normal range". In the US about one third of people have birthweights of around seven pounds or less, and this is one definition of people who are especially vulnerable to later disease. If they happen to know that they did not thrive well after birth and were thin or short at around two years of age, or that their fatness increased rapidly after that age, they should regard themselves as being yet more vulnerable. In the US few people have detailed records of how they grew after birth, but in some European and South American countries each person has a card recording their heights and weights at different ages through childhood.

In the US about one third of people have birthweights of around seven pounds or less, and this is one definition of people who are especially vulnerable to later disease.

"Low birth weight" people need protection from harmful influences that are of lesser or even no consequence to other people. The concept of vulnerable people is familiar. People with thin bones benefit from exercise regimes that enhance bone density. For other people, with denser bones, there may be no benefit. The critical benefits of exercise are different for different people; for some it benefits the bones, for others it benefits the heart, or reduces weight, or lifts the mood.

"Low birth weight" people need protection from harmful influences that are of lesser or even no consequence to other people.

The dawning, but in retrospect obvious, realisation that early development is overwhelmingly important for many aspects of life beyond physical health, is leading to new kinds of study. There is mounting evidence that early growth is linked to the mental, material and social aspects of well-being. In the Helsinki studies people who had low weight gain during infancy did less well at school and had less successful careers and lower incomes in later life. This held

There is mounting evidence that early growth is linked to the mental, material and social aspects of well-being.

whether they were born rich or poor. If they were poor as adults men who had low birthweight were more likely to suffer ill-health than men with higher birthweights. Men who had low birthweight were less likely to get married. More people with low birthweight suffer from depression. Clearly many aspects of well-being beyond the absence of physical illness are linked to low birthweight, and as further research uncovers these, people who had low birthweight will be better able to understand their vulnerabilities.

WHAT CAN PEOPLE WHO HAD LOW BIRTHWEIGHT DO?

Many of us were told as children that success in life comes from the way you play the cards life deals you. How does one identify the cards linked to well-being and longevity? Some of the cards were dealt during development while others were dealt through experience in later childhood and adult life. In so far as your doctor can measure risk factors for disease such as high blood pressure or thin bones a routine medical examination is useful. One outcome may be the prescription of medication to lower blood pressure or strengthen bones. Obviously this is encouraged by the pharmaceutical industry; but neither the pharmaceutical companies nor your doctor can answer the question you may reasonably ask them. "Although trials of your drug have shown that it prolongs the lives of 20 percent of people that take it, will the drug prolong my life?" Every doctor knows that some people respond to a particular medicine while others with the same condition do not. Black Americans with hypertension do not respond to a group of drugs known as "ace-inhibitors". Remarkably little is known about this. To say "it must be genetic" is merely to dismiss it. High blood pressure and diabetes are not the products of a single path of sub-optimal development but of several. Each path may lead to disease through a different process. Each process is likely to respond to different medication.

A clean bill of health at a medical check-up does not equate with well-being. One of the best predictors of the health of a man or woman aged 65 years is the answer to the simple question "Do you feel well?" A positive answer predicts better health for the next twenty years. Your own feelings of well-being predict your future health over and above any measurements your doctor can make. A hope, a reasonable expectation even, is that as knowledge accumulates it will be possible to identify a package of measures which will encompass physical, mental, material and social aspects and will improve well-being, not for the population as a whole, but for you; for each individual has different biological needs, and what is important for you may be unimportant for your neighbor.

Your own feelings of well-being predict your future health over and above any measurements your doctor can make.

PREDICTORS OF VULNERABILITY IN LATER LIFE

Being male. In the US men have shorter lives than women. They die at higher rates at every stage of life: in the womb, during infancy, at every age in childhood and at every age in adult life. The reasons are biological rather than social. The greater vulnerability of male animals was discussed in Chapter 4.

Being non-white. Non-whites in the US live on average for five fewer years than whites. African-Americans are more prone to hypertension and stroke than whites. Native Americans and Hispanics are more prone to diabetes. White women are more prone to hip fractures and breast cancer than black women. Why these differences exist is not known. However babies born to ethnic minorities tend to be smaller than white babies; they tend to grow more slowly during infancy; and many gain weight rapidly after the age of two.

Low educational achievement. A constant finding in surveys of the middle-aged and elderly is that people who achieved less in school get more heart disease and stroke and have shorter lives. People who dropped out of high school live for at least ten years less than people who went to college. Each progressive increase in educational attainment seems to be linked to an increase in lifespan. This defies any simple explanation. It is a feature of European countries as well, and of course within everyone's personal experience there are many exceptions. It is not due to people who stay in school for longer being better taught about healthy life-styles. Though the life-styles of less well educated people do tend to be less healthy, this goes only a small way to explaining their shortened lives. The ability to benefit from education may be a manifestation of general fitness, conferred during early development, and separately linked to better mental function, and to more effective body maintenance and repair.

> *The ability to benefit from education may be a manifestation of general fitness, conferred during early development...*

Low employment status. Men and women in more lowly-paid jobs have shorter, less healthy lives. This is not the product of worse health care. It also applies in European countries where the costs of health care are paid for by the government. European men in lower socio-economic groups live shorter lives. This has been the subject of government reports and recommendations for more than a century. It has persisted despite changes in the main causes of death, from rheumatic heart disease to coronary heart disease, from tuberculosis to asthma. Because, by world standards, poorer people in the US are relatively rich, current ideas focus on the stress of having a low position in the social hierarchy. A low position in a hierarchy may be stressful because there is less control over day-to-day life, less self-esteem and a lesser ability to make decisions about the future. People who had low

> *People who had low birthweight are more vulnerable to stress, and more vulnerable to the ill-health associated with low occupational status.*

birthweight are more vulnerable to stress, and more vulnerable to the ill-health associated with low occupational status

A disease runs in the family. Heart disease, stroke, diabetes and other common diseases tend to run in families, more often in the mother's family than the father's. This has fuelled the search for genes as causes of these disorders. The search has discovered much less than was hoped and it is becoming apparent that the agenda is more complex than the simple passage of genes from one generation to the next. A woman who was born with low birthweight will not only tend to have the chronic illnesses associated with this, but she will tend to have low birthweight babies who in turn will have the same health problems.

> *A woman who was born with low birthweight will not only tend to have the chronic illnesses associated with this, but she will tend to have low birthweight babies who in turn will have the same health problems.*

A poorly nourished mother. The egg from which you were created was laid down while your mother was in her mother's womb. You lived for 20 years or more as a "pre-zygotic" cell, before your father's genes became incorporated into your being. There is plenty of evidence in animals, though little as yet in humans, that the quality of the egg, and hence the quality of the individual to which it will give rise, is affected by the mother's nutrition as an infant, child, adolescent and young woman. Most of us know little about our mother's nutritional state through her life but we do know if she is tall or short, whether or not she grew up in a part of the country where food was abundant and varied, and whether her family was wealthy or not. The children of mothers of short stature, who grew up poor, perhaps during the depression or in one of the poorer states, are at increased risk of chronic disease. How large this effect is we do not yet know; but the next chapter offers a striking example.

> *The children of mothers of short stature, who grew up poor, perhaps during the depression or in one of the poorer states, are at increased risk of chronic disease.*

For people who had low birthweight the presence of one or more of these six predictors of vulnerability may reinforce their wish to protect their health. There are a number of ways in which they can take action.

REGULAR MEDICAL TESTS

Blood pressure. Until middle age people who had low birth weight have only a small increase in blood pressure, too small to be identified as abnormal at a medical check-up. What distinguishes people who had low birthweight from others is that, eventually, they are more likely to develop hypertension, raised blood pressure at a level that requires medication. One explanation of this, described in Chapter 5, is that people who had low birth weight have fewer of the working units, nephrons, in their kidneys, which control blood pressure. For much of a lifetime the kidney is able to compensate for this. However, nephrons die as the body ages: the number falls progressively from an average of around one million per kidney at birth to around a quarter of a million at age 70 years. As this occurs it becomes impossible for people who had low birthweight to maintain their blood pressure within normal limits.

There are other possible processes by which low birthweight may initiate hypertension. People who had low birthweight should have their blood pressure checked regularly; say every two years between 20 and 50 years of age and yearly thereafter. If their blood pressure is above 140/90 they should, in the first instance, change their lifestyle. Loss of around 10 pounds of body weight and reducing alcohol consumption to two drinks a day works for some people: increased physical exercise, stress avoidance and salt restriction works for others. Lifestyle changes are usually unable to stem the rise in blood

> *People who had low birthweight should have their blood pressure checked regularly; say every two years between 20 and 50 years of age and yearly thereafter.*

pressure for more than a few years and medication is likely to be required. As a group, people with hypertension who had low birthweight are more resistant to treatment than people with high birthweight. They are more likely to require a combination of medicines. Once begun, treatment needs to be monitored. The American Heart Association estimates that among the 35 million Americans who know they have high blood pressure only 10 million are taking the right medication in the correct way!

As a group, people with hypertension who had low birthweight are more resistant to treatment than people with high birthweight.

Blood sugar. People who had low birthweight are prone to developing type 2 diabetes. From childhood onwards they tend to be resistant to the effects of the insulin their body makes and they are therefore more likely to develop high sugar levels in their blood. Sugar spills out through the kidneys and can be detected in the urine. Low birthweight people develop diabetes at levels of overweight, defined by body mass index, which may be unimportant to other people. Their ability to maintain normal blood sugar levels is compromised by their resistance to insulin, and this resistance is aggravated by even modest levels of overweight. People from the Indian sub-continent tend to be markedly resistant to insulin, which may reflect their exceptionally low birthweight, around 6 pounds on average. They develop diabetes at young ages, thirty years or less even, and they do so at levels of fatness which are below the average across North America. After the age of forty years people who had low birthweight may wish to have their blood sugars checked at the same time as they have their blood pressure checked. If they are Native American, Hispanic or from the Indian sub-continent these regular checks should begin at thirty years, or earlier if they are overweight or if other family members have diabetes.

After the age of forty years people who had low birthweight may wish to have their blood sugars checked at the same time as they have their blood pressure checked.

Cholesterol. Chapter 8 described how the way the body handles cholesterol is set soon after birth, the time when the liver, which makes and breaks down cholesterol is developing, and when our mothers challenged the system with the high cholesterol content of their breast milk. The links between low birthweight and later cholesterol levels are less clear than those with hypertension and diabetes, but people with low birthweight are more likely to require lipid-lowering medication. There is a clear link between raised cholesterol and slow growth during infancy. Therefore, people who had low birthweight may wish to have regular checks of blood cholesterol, both the total amount and its two main components, HDL and non-HDL cholesterol.

> *Therefore, people who had low birthweight may wish to have regular checks of blood cholesterol, both the total amount and its two main components, HDL and non-HDL cholesterol.*

MUSCLE AND BONE STRENGTH

Muscularity and fitness. Slow growth in the womb and during the first few months after birth is accompanied by a reduction in the amount of muscle that is laid down. People who had low birthweight tend to have low muscle mass through their lives. In later life their weakness can be measured by the reduced strength of their hand grip; and by their being readily fatigued by simple repetitive movements. They are less fit, a term which includes the body's strength, flexibility and endurance. Within a group of people, the least fit have at least twice the death rates at each age as do the fittest. It is a graded relationship. Regular physical exercise increases fitness, reduces the risk of heart disease and counteracts the development of obesity and resistance to insulin. It makes muscles stronger and more efficient.

> *People who had low birthweight tend to have low muscle mass through their lives.*

Among the kinds of exercise, sports such as tennis, basketball, squash and swimming have a strong effect on strength, flexibility and endurance. So too does housework! Gardening and golf benefit all these three aspects of fitness, but less strongly. A brisk walk for 30 minutes three times a week brings measurable though modest benefits for strength and flexibility. To improve health by becoming fitter requires aerobic physical activity. This is defined as activity which can be sustained for at least 12 minutes without a break, because the muscles are receiving oxygen and energy from the circulating blood. In contrast, during anaerobic activities, such as carrying heavy loads, the blood is not able to supply the oxygen and energy required and the muscles have to use different chemical processes to obtain energy. These processes cannot be sustained for long. A generally agreed recommendation is that aerobic exercise should be sufficiently intense to cause sweating. Intermittent exercise such as housework is as effective as sustained exercise over the same period. Therefore, a routine which incorporates parking the car a few blocks from the office, using stairs where possible, a walk at lunchtime, gardening at weekends can, it seems, be as effective as an aerobics class, swimming and the gym.

Bone strength. The strength of a bone depends on its size and the density of the calcium salts within it. This 'bone mass' reaches a peak in early adult life and thereafter gradually declines. The risk of an osteoporotic fracture depends on the peak bone mass attained

Low birthweight babies have a lower bone mass which persists throughout their lives.

and the subsequent rate of loss. Low birthweight babies have a lower bone mass which persists throughout their lives. People who were small at birth or who did not thrive during infancy also have life-long alterations in two hormones, growth hormone and cortisol, which influence bone mass. These alterations lead both to lower peak bone mass and to more rapid loss of bone mass with age.

People who had low birthweight, especially women, may benefit from three actions that help to prevent osteoporosis. Regular weight-bearing exercise, as described in the previous section; consuming milk and dairy products, which are rich in calcium; and avoiding smoking and excess alcohol consumption, which are toxic to bone.

AVOIDING FATNESS

Although low birth weight does not predispose to obesity, people who had low birth weight tend to store fat in different parts of the body. If they become obese they tend to be 'centrally' obese, with fat stored on the trunk and abdomen rather than on the hips and limbs. People with central obesity are prone to hypertension and diabetes.

> *Although low birth weight does not predispose to obesity, people who had low birth weight tend to store fat in different parts of the body.*

Children who are born thin and remain thin for the first two years, or children who become thin after birth, tend to have an early 'adiposity rebound', as was described in the last chapter. This predisposes to overweight and obesity in adult life. If people who had low birthweight become overweight or obese they not only tend to be centrally obese but they are less able to tolerate it. At any level of overweight or obesity people who had low birthweight are more likely to develop diabetes than people with higher birthweights.

DIET

People who had low birthweight or grew slowly during infancy may have a reduced capacity to refashion food (Chapter 6). It follows that their diets should have a high 'goodness of fit' to their needs. Our understanding of this is seriously incomplete and advice today cannot go beyond stressing the importance of a varied diet, to provide the nutrients that the body is unable to make for itself. Recent research shows that, in people with low birthweight, diets high in saturated fat may more readily reduce the amount of the beneficial form of cholesterol, HDL cholesterol, in the blood. The evidence supporting this is not conclusive, and is partly based on studies in animals; but prudence suggests that avoidance of foods high in saturated fat may be especially relevant to people with low birthweight. These people also have a reduced functional capacity in their kidneys. One of the main functions of the kidney is to maintain the body's balance of salt. Excessive salt is linked to high blood pressure. Since the average American eats at least twice as much salt as his or her body requires people who had low birthweight should be cautious about their intakes of processed foods.

HANDLING STRESS

When people feel threatened they respond by activating particular nervous pathways and by releasing hormones, including adrenaline and cortisol. These "stress" responses occur in all mammals and help us to survive. However, each year some seven million Americans consult their doctors because they have symptoms of stress, which include anxiety and depression. Stress has been linked to a range of physical illnesses including heart disease and diabetes.

People who had low birthweight have heightened responses to stress. We do not yet know whether this is important for their health

People who had low birthweight have heightened responses to stress.

but the balance of evidence suggests that it is. Therefore if they develop symptoms of chronic stress their need for professional advice may be more pressing than that of other people. The key symptoms are constantly feeling tense or on edge, feeling irritable, difficulty in concentrating or making decisions, difficulty in relaxing or sleeping, and recurrent headaches.

SUMMARY

The places where life expectancy is longest are those where people are not only healthier but biologically younger. 75 year old people may be biologically similar to 65 year old people in less healthy places. There are two challenges in later life. One is to avoid age-related diseases, which include heart disease and diabetes: the other is to slow the rate of biological aging. The two challenges are linked but disease is not an inevitable consequence of aging. In later life people who had low birthweight are both at increased risk of disease and are more frail. There are a number of ways in which they can protect themselves.

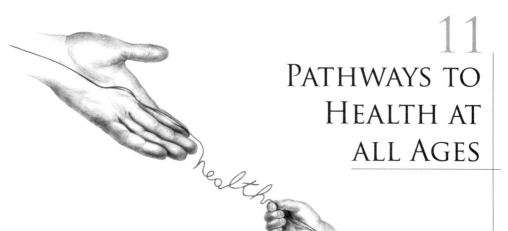

11
PATHWAYS TO HEALTH AT ALL AGES

HEART DISEASE, STROKE, DIABETES, hypertension, osteoporosis, the most common causes of human illness and death, originate in two universal phenomena. The first is plasticity during development; the way each individual responds to the conditions in which he or she develops before and after birth. Malnutrition during development has costs: for humans these are premature disability and death. The second phenomenon is compensatory growth, the ability to grow rapidly following a period of malnutrition and slowing of growth. Few living things grow as fast as they can because the costs of rapid growth are not worth paying: for humans the cost of rapid increase in fatness after the age of two years is chronic disease in late life.

> Malnutrition during development has costs: for humans these are premature disability and death.

To those who have become accustomed to the viewpoint that disease is the price of bad genes and bad living, this new perspective may seem implausible. But what at first sight seems implausible often turns out to be the way things are. In the fall the Arctic Tern leaves the tundra

> …this new perspective may seem implausible. But what at first sight seems implausible often turns out to be the way things are.

157

within the Arctic Circle where it breeds, and flies down to the edge of the Antarctic ice-pack where it spends the winter, before flying back to the Arctic the following summer. It flies 21,000 miles each year, roughly the circumference of the earth. It is unbelievable: but it happens to be true. Before you read this book did you know that well-intentioned attempts to give impoverished mothers more protein resulted in smaller babies; or that feeding orphan Indian girls disrupted their sexual physiology; or that ewes give birth to bigger lambs if they are starved in mid-pregnancy?

OUT OF TOUCH WITH NATURE

A hundred years ago many American children were stunted and thin and large numbers died, of infective illnesses and poor nutrition. To remedy this, sanitation and hygiene were improved, overcrowding in the home was reduced, more food became available, and children were no longer employed in factories. Soon children grew faster and became bigger, and fewer died. Surely this is a triumph of public health? That fewer died must be a triumph, but why is it good to have larger children? The American public health physician René Dubos wrote that "one of the criteria of health most widely accepted at the present time is that children should grow as large and as fast as possible. But is size such a desirable attribute? Is the bigger child happier? Will he contribute more to man's cultural heritage? Or does his larger size merely mean that he will need a larger motor car, become a larger soldier, and in his turn beget still larger children? The criteria of growth developed for the production of market pigs would hardly be adequate for animals feeding on acorns in the forests and fending for themselves as free individuals. Nor are they for men. Size and weight are not desirable in themselves and their relation to health and happiness is at most obscure."

Human well-being is finely balanced. In exchange for a few centimeters increase in height, we have perturbed our reproductive biology. In 1959, an editorial in the Lancet remarked that it was becoming difficult to find choirboys. The race to an earlier puberty left too little pre-pubertal life in which musical skills could develop. The boys' voices had broken before they could be fully trained. Such changes happen over several generations and we come to accept them. What is overlooked, perhaps, is the message they bring. During development the human body is highly sensitive. Without intending to we have shortened childhood, by several years. The body is sensitive because that is how its systems function. These systems are tailored to meet the baby's particular needs at a particular time. Somewhere in this tailoring lie the origins of lifelong health.

> *Human well-being is finely balanced. In exchange for a few centimeters increase in height, we have perturbed our repro- ductive biology.*

> *Without intending to we have shortened childhood, by several years.*

Now that more food is available, small babies in western countries and in the cities of the Third World are able to compensate by rapidly putting on weight. It is 'normal' in that it is a biological response that has been passed down to us through our genes, and has required a change in circumstances to be evoked. It is becoming 'usual'. But is it optimal? Or is it leading to heart disease and diabetes ? We have created the conditions in which epidemics of these diseases are occurring. We need to manage the growth of our children. The American 'escape from hunger' is indeed a triumph, but we need to address its costs.

> *We need to manage the growth of our children.*

We need to understand how our biology is changing and why better nutrition has created disease. Long ago, the pathologist Virchow wrote, "disease is life under changed conditions." Ordinary people in the US have never been in a better position to bestow upon their babies resilient bodies that will withstand the assaults of the external environment through their lives. We have improved children's nutrition, and lifespan has increased by forty years within no more than a century. We now need to deal with some unwanted and unforeseen consequences of this achievement.

Unfortunately we have lost touch with the natural world. Heart disease appeared in our midst, a new disease. We took refuge in

> *Unfortunately we have lost touch with the natural world.*

simplistic ideas: too much milk; too many pizzas; too many cigarettes. Smoking is a considerable insult to the body; but when the last cigarette has been thrown away, there will still be heart disease and diabetes, and osteoporosis and breast cancer and the other diseases that arise out of changes in our biological systems as we develop. What constitutes a varied and balanced diet has been widely agreed in the US for almost one hundred years. Within broad guidelines there are many choices, determined by levels of activity, body size and preferences. But, removed from agriculture and the land, people today have lost confidence in their ability to make good food choices. They seek prescription, not freedom of choice. They want to be told for how many minutes they should exercise each day, how much milk to drink, how many portions of fruit. Pregnancy books give table upon table of how much of each nutrient there is in each food, how many portions are desirable. Yet there are countless different ways in which a woman can negotiate the dietary needs of pregnancy.

The diets of previous generations who lived on the rich farmlands of the Middle Atlantic States, or on the west coast, would not have been greatly enhanced had they had access to modern nutritional knowledge. Science does not make good diets better. The Mediterranean diet was not invented in a laboratory. The triumphs of nutritional science have been in rescuing people from dietary deficiencies created by human society: from rickets in the slums of cities; from pellagra in the southern states; from protein-calorie deficiency in the Third World. Most Americans have access to rich farmlands through their local supermarket; but cut off from tradition, and lacking the requisite simple knowledge, they are making bad food choices.

In human societies customs which fly in the face of nature readily take root. The French realized long ago that, needing strong young men for their weakened armies, they had to protect girls and young women, the mothers of the future. Every farmer knows the importance of protecting female animals for the benefit of the next generation. Yet across Asia feeding the boy child is given priority over feeding the girl, and the newly married wife is the last member of the family to eat. Many young women in western countries aspire to be thin, and they diet to shrink themselves. Now even pregnant women are dieting. But in other animals large size and well-developed sexual characteristics demonstrate biological fitness, the ability to reproduce successfully. Why do some young western women wish to show themselves as less fit? Why do others want to pretend to be fitter than they are, having surgery to make large breasts larger still? We need to find a better way.

We have created the junk food industry for our children. The typical American eats three hamburgers and four orders of French fries every week. Never was it easier for a two year old child to put on weight rapidly. Increase in fatness is commanded by an increased appetite, which is satisfied by nutritionally inadequate, but highly palatable, processed food. This in turn generates a continuing appetite—for junk food. We are not seeking a return to Arcadia, to a past of sturdy peasants. In America there never was one. They, the government, cannot help. Each family has to make its own food decisions because each family is different.

PATHWAYS TO DISEASE

Darwin recognized that the fittest people, those who survive and reproduce, are those who are best adapted to their surroundings, the external environment. The French physiologist Claude Bernard realized that fitness depends on the interplay between the internal and external environment. The fittest people are those best able to resist the impact of the outside world, and maintain constancy within their bodies. The internal environment is established during development, through responses to nutrition and other stimuli from the external environment. Through our lives our internal environment modulates our responses to the conditions in which we live. We know that our early experiences of measles, chickenpox or mumps, condition our responses to the viruses when we again encounter them. This is an example of a general phenomenon whereby early experiences condition responses in later life. This is what underlies chronic disease. The men in Helsinki who grew well in the womb are now indifferent to poor living conditions, at least in so far as these predispose to heart disease.

The fittest people are those best able to resist the impact of the outside world, and maintain constancy within their bodies.

Disease does not have a single cause. The tubercle bacillus is necessary for the development of tuberculosis. The discovery of this bacillus encouraged the idea that for each disease there is a single cause. But in the past tubercle bacilli were everywhere, and who became sick and died, and who met the bacteria's challenge and became forever resistant to it, was determined by their nutritional state, their internal environment. Now geneticists look for single causes, "the gene for heart disease". There is no single gene; there are many and what they do depends on what is happening elsewhere in the body. Genes do one thing in one person and another thing in another. They are part of a democracy.

A well-known entertainer died recently. His widow wrote that he died "from an entirely random disease, neither hereditary nor caused by lifestyle." But the essence of chronic disease is not a single, overwhelming disruption of the body occurring either at conception or in middle age. There are pathways to disease. Life is like a game of pinball. The ball is launched by a spring; it strikes a pin projecting from the surface of the table; it is deflected according to the speed and direction from which it came. The pin's effect on the ball is conditioned by what has gone before, by the way the spring launched the ball. The ball moves on until it strikes another pin, which pin it strikes is determined by what has gone before, on how it was deflected by the previous pin. Eventually it disappears down a tunnel having amassed a score, depending on which pins it has struck. Health through a lifetime is launched by the mother and a strong launch in the womb goes a long way to ensuring a good score. The well-grown baby becomes vulnerable if it fails to thrive in infancy. But if it thrives it can withstand rapid weight gain and poor living conditions in childhood and adult life and reach old age in good health. A weak launch and poor growth in the womb, leaves the baby vulnerable. Low scoring pins await it—rapid childhood weight gain, poor living conditions. It is not doomed, but it is vulnerable.

Life is like a game of pinball.

Health through a lifetime is launched by the mother and a strong launch in the womb goes a long way to ensuring a good score.

THE FAILURE OF MEDICAL RESEARCH

Medical research has had many successes, the control of infectious disease, elimination of dietary deficiencies, antibiotics, the treatment of chronic disease. Which is why our current failure to prevent chronic disease is surprising. Over half a century we, the medical research community, have made little progress in stemming the epidemic of chronic disease. At the start we looked only for simple answers. Too much of one food in the diet, too little of another:

this has not worked out as a basis for effective prevention. We did identify an enemy, smoking, but this is not the key. We borrowed a model of disease that is appropriate to rare inherited disorders, and hoped it would work for common disease. It did not. So we are reduced to being spectators. In the US we watch as stroke declines. We do not understand why it is happening, though we take the credit. Diabetes and obesity are rising. We do not know why, but we blame it on the bad habits of the sufferers. Breast cancer is rising: we can do nothing to allay this. It has been surprisingly easy for us as scientists to remain engaged with governments on the basis that our research might, just possibly might, one day, prevent disease. They give us more money and we give them more of the same. In Public Health there have been more displays of activity than demonstrations of effectiveness. While people perish legislators debate whether it is lawful to smoke in your car with the windows open!

One reason why we have been able to sustain our fruitless quest is that research has undoubtedly improved the clinical care of patients, which gives us credibility. Many patients now survive who would previously have died and I, like all doctors, would like to claim a tiny share of the credit for this. The trouble is that, while patients are grateful for new drugs and operations, what they really want is not to be patients at all. In this we are failing them.

> *...while patients are grateful for new drugs and operations what they really want is not to be patients at all.*

The idea that heart disease, stroke, diabetes, osteoporosis are disorders of development, has been supported by three groups of people: the general public, biologists and some doctors. For 'reductionist' scientists who devote their time to studying some fragment of the human body, an obstacle to embracing these new ideas has simply been a lack of understanding of how their particular fragment fits into the jigsaw that is now being put together.

There are glaring gaps in our knowledge. Research could readily fill them. We do not know, for example, how a mother's diet at the time she conceives affects the growth of her baby. This can easily be addressed. We know a lot about it in sheep, pigs, cows and horses, because breeding domestic animals is a major industry. We do not know why rapid increase in fatness during childhood leads to later disease. Much is known about this in farm animals.

The public wants more research on these themes in humans. Thousands of them are helping in studies around the world. They are not sick and have little to gain personally. For no financial reward they give their time, submit to intimate measurements and blood tests: some even spend days and nights in hospital. To them it is obvious that good paths of early growth and development are the greatest gift society can give to the next generation.

> *...good paths of early growth and development are the greatest gift society can give to the next generation.*

WHY BILL CLINTON HAD A HEART ATTACK

So why did the slim, physically active former president, Bill Clinton, who did not smoke cigarettes, come so close to death in September 2004? He was born in a small town in southwest Arkansas. In 1946, while his mother was in the 25th week of her pregnancy, his father was returning home from Chicago when a tire on his car burst and he lost control. He died by the roadside. "I was born on my grandfather's birthday, a couple of weeks early, weighing in at a respectable six pounds eight ounces, on a twenty-one inch frame," he writes in his autobiography. Twenty-one inches is a long baby, well above the average for the US and for even the world's tallest populations, such as the Scandinavians. But six pounds eight ounces is not a heavy baby. It is well below the average for the US, but around the average for countries such as India and Thailand. Compared with someone who weighed nine pounds at birth a man or women who weighed six pounds has a twenty-five percent higher risk of heart disease and a thirty percent higher risk of stroke. The president was also thin when he was born. He would have lacked muscle, for which the most critical period of development is before birth. The development of his liver, which was about to learn how to handle the high cholesterol diet in his mother's milk, is likely to have been impaired.

A year or so after he was born he was left in the care of his grandmother, his mother's mother, Edith Cassidy, known as Mammaw. "Mammaw's main goals for me were that I would eat a lot, learn a lot, and always be neat and clean... She also stuffed me at every meal, because conventional wisdom at the time was that a fat baby was a healthy one, as long as he bathed every day." Having been born thin, lacking muscle, the future President was putting on weight rapidly in the early years after weaning. This is likely to have given him a body with a low ratio of muscle to fat, a body composition known to be linked to heart disease in later life.

His candid descriptions of childhood repeatedly refer to his lack of athleticism, which can be attributed to his lack of muscular development before birth. When he was 5 he broke his leg trying to jump over a rope in the school playground. "The kids would line up on one side and take turns running and jumping over it. All the other kids cleared the rope. Me, I didn't clear the rope. I was a little chunky anyway, and slow..."

Bill Clinton seems to have followed one of the pathways of growth which lead to later disease. In his particular game of pinball the ball had a weak launch, and then struck the low-scoring pin of rapid childhood weight gain. He was thin at birth either because of events during the pregnancy, or because of his mother's own growth in the womb. We do not know to what extent stressful events in pregnancy, such as bereavement, prejudice a mother's ability to nourish her baby, but there is plenty of evidence that they do. It seems likely that his mother was not well nourished in the womb. Her own mother, whom the President describes as a "poor white southern woman", was only five foot tall. The story of his illness matches the recent conclusions of the National Institute of Health in Washington. "Coronary heart disease, the number one cause of death in adult men and women, is more closely related to low birth weight than to known behavioral risk factors. Thus, a significant portion of the disease burden borne by adults may have roots in antenatal nutrition and a poor transgenerational maternal health history." The thesis of this book is that the origins of heart attacks do not lie in manslaughter by burgers and barbecued ribs, but in an unforeseen consequence of the American dream, the ascent from poverty.

> *The thesis of this book is that the origins of heart attacks do not lie in manslaughter by burgers and barbecued ribs, but in an unforeseen consequence of the American dream...*

FROM HUNGER TO PLENTY

Because so many children die in Third World countries they have been the focus of attention by international agencies such as UNICEF, the World Bank and the World Health Organization. Increasingly, however, it is becoming apparent that the focus of attention should move to the mother and infant. There is a double burden in the Third World, undernutrition and excess nutrition. Both are rooted in poverty. Both are forms of malnutrition, and they co-exist in the same communities, even in the same households. The United Nations Standing Committee on Nutrition, has written, "...this double burden of malnutrition has common causes, inadequate fetal and infant and young child nutrition followed by exposure (including through marketing practices) to unhealthy energy dense nutrient poor foods and lack of physical activity. The window

> *There is a double burden in the Third World, undernutrition and excess nutrition.*

of opportunity lies from pre-pregnancy to around twenty-four months of a child's age."

The world epidemics of heart disease and diabetes are being driven by this double burden. In order to improve the nutrition of babies another issue has to be confronted. Across most of Asia and much of North Africa, death rates among women are much higher than would be expected from the death rates among men. Since, given the same nutrition and health care, women generally have lower death rates than men, this suggests that women are being neglected. There are an estimated one hundred million fewer women in the world than there should be, given the number of men—37 million fewer in India, 44 million in China. Three components of the neglect of women have been identified. First, girls are given less food than boys and are less likely to receive health care if they are sick. Second, young women of reproductive age are thin because they are undernourished. As a consequence of this many babies are born with low birthweight: 20 percent of babies born in South Asia in the year 2000 weighed less than 5½ pounds (2.5 kg). In California, babies may be considered for intensive care if they weigh less than 6 pounds (2.7 kg), which would apply to more than half of all babies born in India! Finally, in later life women have high rates of disorders known to be the result of malnutrition—recurrent illness and inability to do physical work. Among both men and women, death rates from heart disease, stroke and high blood pressure are higher in South Asia than in any western country.

> *The world epidemics of heart disease and diabetes are being driven by this double burden.*

The intense concern with this issue among doctors and health workers in Asia is evident from the flourishing programs of research there. The first world conference on the themes of this book was not held in the US or Europe, but in India. International concern is rising, but the agencies grapple with politics. They are necessarily diverted into handling crises such as AIDS, and become distracted by taking on issues such as smoking which, though damaging, does not lie at the heart of human well-being.

Underlying the epidemics of heart disease and diabetes that accompany westernization is our inability to improve the nourishment of babies in the womb as rapidly as we can improve the nutrition of children. During the so-called 'nutritional transition' children immediately benefit from the increased availability of food. For the full benefit to reach babies it takes more than one generation, because part of a mother's ability to nourish her baby depends on her refashioning capacity and her nutritional stores, which are the product of her growth and nutrition since her life in the womb. During the period of transition many small babies continue to be born but they are able to increase their fatness rapidly during childhood—a pathway to later disease.

Underlying the epidemics of heart disease and diabetes that accompany westernization is our inability to improve the nourishment of babies in the womb as rapidly as we can improve the nutrition of children.

Experiments in animals have demonstrated that the diet of one generation may affect several generations. A colony of rats was given a diet deficient in protein. When the colony was re-fed with a normal diet it took three generations before fetal growth and development were restored to normal. It follows that as women in places such as India, China, North Africa, South America cease to be chronically malnourished and no longer carry out heavy manual labor during pregnancy, it will take more than one generation before the full benefits reach the baby. India underwent the 'Green Revolution' during 1967 to 1978. Expansion of farmland and improvements in farming practices increased the availability of food and abolished large-scale famine. Nevertheless the average birthweight in India remains around six pounds. Similarly, for people who emigrate to western countries from poorly nourished communities, Mexican migrants to the US for example, more than one generation will be required before the growth of their babies improves to the level of the host country.

Genevieve Stearns, a nutritionist at the University of Iowa, has summarized the position as follows. "The best provision for well-being in any period of life is to arrive at that point in good nutritional and physical status. The well-born infant is sturdier throughout infancy than the baby poorly born; the sturdy infant has stores to give impetus to growth in the pre-school years. The child who is in excellent nutrition will have stores to be drawn upon during the rapid growth of puberty. The well-nourished mother can nourish her fetus well; therefore the best insurance for a healthy infant is a mother who is healthy and well-nourished throughout her entire life, as well as during the period of pregnancy itself."

From this it follows that during the nutritional transition, the nourishment of girls and young women should be the highest priority...

From this it follows that during the nutritional transition the nourishment of girls and young women should be the highest priority, as it was in France. Neglecting this in favor of older people or boys and young men sets the stage for outbreaks of heart disease and diabetes.

MOTHERS CAN BE CONFIDENT

For so long as the main aim of pregnancy has been the avoidance of disaster, a dead or deformed baby, a mother may feel that she will be to blame if things go wrong. She must have neglected to eat something essential or have eaten too much of something harmful. And so mothers have taken refuge in prescriptive pregnancy guides that set out the nutrient content of each food—which vitamins, which minerals, how much of each—and recommend the amount of each food, and the size of the portions. We do not use such prescriptions for our children's diets after birth. We offer variety and balance and recognize that the demands of physical exercise and growth differ from one child to another. Each child develops along a unique path, both before and after birth, and its needs cannot be met by formulas, as though it were a machine. The plane that will take me from Portland to Dallas tomorrow is the product of precise design and an inflexible maintenance routine. It makes the journey twice a day according to a tight timetable. Hundreds of thousands of migratory birds make the same journey each year, but they are prepared by nature, guided by instinct and fly to a timetable determined by sunshine, wind and weather.

Today in the western world mothers should trust nature and enter pregnancy with confidence. They are the custodians of a marvellous system handed down to them through millions of years of evolution. Natural selection has honed the system for success. Growth and survival of the baby is a centerpiece of evolutionary strategy. Most of the process is controlled by nature: the egg's journey to the womb, the embryo's implantation, the growth of the placenta, all occur without a mother's knowledge. The long and complex supply line which brings food from the mother to the baby develops without her consent. She is the arena for nature's performance and all she can do is acquiesce. If we protect the health and nutrition of girls and young women we can make an end to heart disease and diabetes. Each year the lives of millions of people will be spared. Many more will be saved from chronic ill health.

CHART 1

Height in feet & inches	Weight in pounds																Height in cm
	21	28	35	42	49	56	63	70	77	84	91	98	105	112	119	126	
2'11"	12	16	20	24	28	32	36	40	44	48	52	56	60	64	68	72	89
2'12"	11	15	19	23	27	30	34	38	42	46	49	53	57	61	65	68	91
3'1"	11	14	18	22	25	29	32	36	40	43	47	50	54	58	61	65	94
3'2"	10	14	17	20	24	27	31	34	37	41	44	48	51	55	58	61	97
3'3"	10	13	16	19	23	26	29	32	36	39	42	45	49	52	55	58	99
3'4"	9	12	15	18	22	25	28	31	34	37	40	43	46	49	52	55	102
3'5"	9	12	15	18	20	23	26	29	32	35	38	41	44	47	50	53	104
3'6"	8	11	14	17	20	22	25	28	31	33	36	39	42	45	47	50	107
3'7"	8	11	13	16	19	21	24	27	29	32	35	37	40	43	45	48	109
3'8"	8	10	13	15	18	20	23	25	28	31	33	36	38	41	43	46	112
3'9"	7	10	12	15	17	19	22	24	27	29	32	34	36	39	41	44	114
3'10"	7	9	12	14	16	19	21	23	26	28	30	33	35	37	40	42	117
3'11"	7	9	11	13	16	18	20	22	25	27	29	31	33	36	38	40	119
3'12"	6	9	11	13	15	17	19	21	23	26	28	30	32	34	36	38	122
4'1"	6	8	10	12	14	16	18	20	23	25	27	29	31	33	35	37	124
4'2"	6	8	10	12	14	16	18	20	22	24	26	28	30	31	33	35	127
4'3"	6	8	9	11	13	15	17	19	21	23	25	26	28	30	32	34	130
4'4"	5	7	9	11	13	15	16	18	20	22	24	25	27	29	31	33	132
4'5"	5	7	9	11	12	14	16	18	19	21	23	25	26	28	30	32	135
4'6"	5	7	8	10	12	14	15	17	19	20	22	24	25	27	29	30	137
4'7"	5	7	8	10	11	13	15	16	18	20	21	23	24	26	28	29	140
4'8"	5	6	8	9	11	13	14	16	17	19	20	22	24	25	27	28	142
4'9"	5	6	8	9	11	12	14	15	17	18	20	21	23	24	26	27	145
4'10"	4	6	7	9	10	12	13	15	16	18	19	20	22	23	25	26	147
4'11"	4	6	7	8	10	11	13	14	16	17	18	20	21	23	24	25	150
4'12"	4	5	7	8	10	11	12	14	15	16	18	19	21	22	23	25	152
5'1"	4	5	7	8	9	11	12	13	15	16	17	19	20	21	22	24	155
5'2"	4	5	6	8	9	10	12	13	14	15	17	18	19	20	22	23	157
5'3"	4	5	6	7	9	10	11	12	14	15	16	17	19	20	21	22	160
	10	13	16	19	22	25	29	32	35	38	41	44	48	51	54	57	

BODY MASS INDEX CALCULATOR FOR CHILDREN OVER 3 YEARS OLD

Weight in kilograms

CHART 2

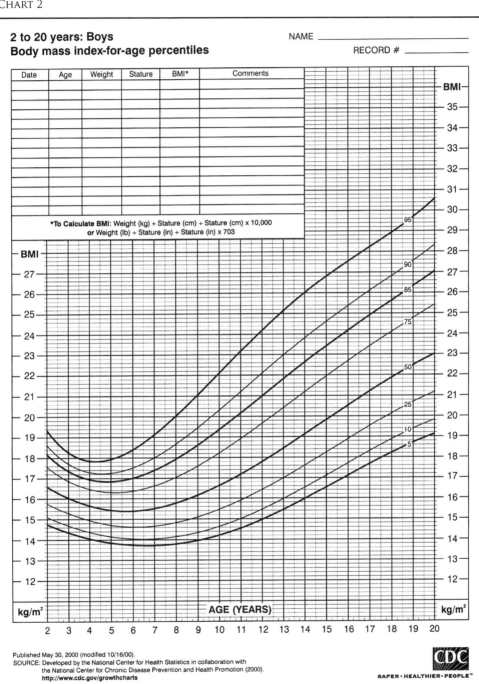

2 to 20 years: Boys
Body mass index-for-age percentiles

NAME _____

RECORD # _____

Date	Age	Weight	Stature	BMI*	Comments

*To Calculate BMI: Weight (kg) ÷ Stature (cm) ÷ Stature (cm) x 10,000
or Weight (lb) ÷ Stature (in) ÷ Stature (in) x 703

BMI

AGE (YEARS)

kg/m²

Published May 30, 2000 (modified 10/16/00).
SOURCE: Developed by the National Center for Health Statistics in collaboration with
the National Center for Chronic Disease Prevention and Health Promotion (2000).
http://www.cdc.gov/growthcharts

CDC
SAFER · HEALTHIER · PEOPLE™

173

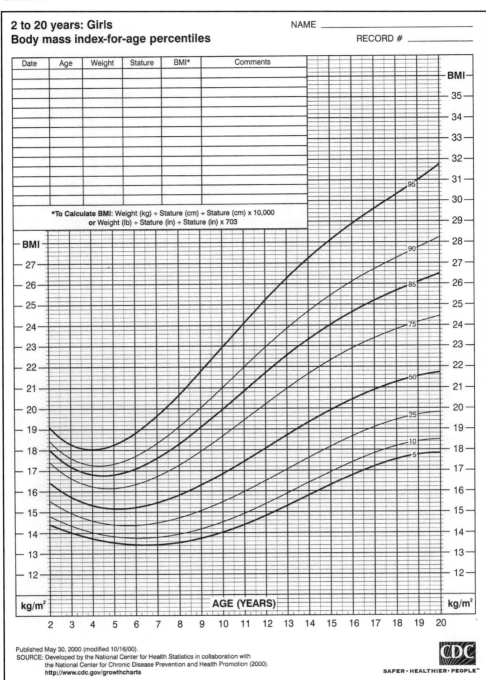

2 to 20 years: Girls
Body mass index-for-age percentiles

NAME _____

RECORD # _____

Date	Age	Weight	Stature	BMI*	Comments

*To Calculate BMI: Weight (kg) ÷ Stature (cm) ÷ Stature (cm) x 10,000
or Weight (lb) ÷ Stature (in) ÷ Stature (in) x 703

AGE (YEARS)

kg/m²

kg/m²

Published May 30, 2000 (modified 10/16/00).
SOURCE: Developed by the National Center for Health Statistics in collaboration with
the National Center for Chronic Disease Prevention and Health Promotion (2000).
http://www.cdc.gov/growthcharts

CDC
SAFER · HEALTHIER · PEOPLE™